Rheumatology Examination and Injection Techniques

Michael Doherty
Professor of Rheumatology, Rheumatology Unit, City Hospital, Nottingham, UK

Brian L Hazleman
Consultant Rheumatologist, Rheumatology Research Unit, Addenbrooke's Hospital, Cambridge, UK

Charles W Hutton
Consultant Rheumatologist, Derriford Hospital, Plymouth, UK

Peter J Maddison
Consultant Rheumatologist, Ysbyty Gwynedd, Bangor, UK

J David Perry
Consultant Rheumatologist, The Royal London Hospital, Whitechapel, London, UK

SECOND EDITION

W. B. SAUNDERS COMPANY LTD

London • Edinburgh • New York • Philadelphia • Toronto • Sydney

W.B. Saunders
An imprint of Harcourt Brace and Company Limited

© 1999 Harcourt Brace and Company Limited
First published 1992

This book is printed on acid free paper.

A catalogue record for this book is available from the British Library

ISBN 0–7020–2387–6

Typeset by J&L Composition Ltd, Filey, North Yorkshire
Printed in Great Britain by Anthony Rowe Ltd, Chippenham, Wiltshire

Contents

Preface   vi

Section 1: Introduction to examination

1. **Introduction**   3
   Michael Doherty

2. **The minimum rheumatological examination**   16
   Michael Doherty

3. **Disease assessment indices and outcome measures**   23
   Brian L Hazleman

Section 2: Examination of specific regions

4. **The shoulder**   31
   Brian L Hazleman

5. **The elbow**   51
   Michael Doherty

6. **The hand**   61
   Charles W Hutton

7. **The spine**   71
   Charles W Hutton

8. **The hip**   86
   Peter J Maddison

9. **The knee**   96
   J David Perry

10. **The foot and ankle**   112
    Peter J Maddison

11. **The temporomandibular joint**   128
    Brian L Hazleman

12. **Posture and gait**   136
    J David Perry

Section 3: Aspiration and injection techniques

13. **Principles of joint aspiration and steroid injection**   147
    Brian L Hazleman

14. **Examination of synovial fluid**   150
    Michael Doherty

Recommended further reading   155
Index   157

A colour plate section appears between pages 156 and 157.

Preface

Rheumatological problems are exceedingly common in the community, may relate to disease in other systems, and are the single most important factor influencing disability in later life. The diagnosis and assessment of arthritis and periarticular lesions is almost entirely dependent on clinical skills and applied knowledge of regional anatomy. Unfortunately such skills are often poorly taught during student and specialist training and many doctors feel less than competent in approaching examination of this large system.

This popular book represents the first combined approach to this topic by UK rheumatologists. The second edition has allowed an expansion of content, and an improvement and increase in the number of illustrations. The book provides an introduction to important principles of the locomotor history and examination, proposes a brief screening procedure for regional localisation of problems, and then covers examination of each region in detail. Throughout, the emphasis is on common periarticular as well as articular abnormalities. Joint aspiration and periarticular/articular injection are common requirements for rheumatological assessment and management, and instruction on these techniques is, therefore, included for each region. A new chapter specifically addresses methods of locomotor disease assessment.

This book is particularly suited to trainess in rheumatology, but is also appropriate for trainee orthopaedic surgeons, general practice trainees and trainers, and interested allied health professionals. In addition the book contains enough detail to be of interest to established consultant rheumatologists.

Introduction to examination

As its name suggests the locomotor system is primarily concerned with movement. The structure of its component tissues reflects this functional requirement, being designed to permit smooth efficient motion between articulating structures, while at the same time restraining and controlling excessive potentially harmful movement.

DEVELOPMENT AND BASIC STRUCTURE OF JOINTS

Bone, cartilage and muscle develop from mesenchymal tissue. Their basic structural features are self-differentiating, the chief aspects of differentiation occurring during the embryonic period (4th to 8th weeks). Mesenchymal tissues around the notochord segment to form primitive vertebrae from which dorsal and lateral projections subsequently form the neural arch and costal processes: occipital segments fuse to form part of the skull, and sacral segments fuse to form part of the pelvis. Limb buds appear in the cervical and lumbar segments and then grow peripherally, the proximal girdles migrating caudally but retaining their cervical nerve connections. By the end of the 8th week the embryo has assumed a recognisable human form, and the remainder of gestation (fetal period) is largely concerned with growth. During this period, and throughout subsequent life, locomotor development is strongly influenced by physical stresses associated with movement. Movement itself is thus one of the controlling forces that adapts the structure and organisation of locomotor tissues. Points worthy of note (particularly in respect of congenital skeletal anomalies) include:

- axial development occurs in a craniad–caudad manner;
- limb buds grow peripherally;
- upper limbs develop a little in advance of lower limbs (insults during the period of limb development affect a more distal portion of the upper extremity than of the lower extremity);

- the number of rays increases distally (one in upper arm and thigh, two in forearm and shin, three in carpus and tarsus, five in hand and foot).

Joints are discontinuities in the skeleton that permit controlled mobility. Their varying structure reflects varying functional requirements. If very little movement is required the bone ends are firmly joined together in a continuous fashion (*synarthrosis*, Fig. 1.1). The two bones may be bridged by either:

- **Fibrous tissue** (*syndesmosis*), permitting almost no motion (e.g. skull sutures, interosseous membrane between radius and ulna), or
- **Cartilage** (*synchondrosis*), usually permitting a limited degree of movement. *Primary* cartilaginous joints, e.g.

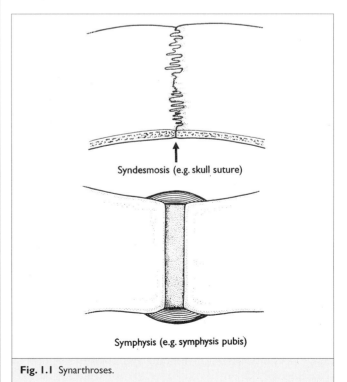

Syndesmosis (e.g. skull suture)

Symphysis (e.g. symphysis pubis)

Fig. 1.1 Synarthroses.

Capsule (thickened
to form ligaments)

Synovium

Fibrocartilage meniscus

Hyaline articular cartilage

Joint cavity

Fig. 1.2 Synovial joints (diarthroses).

between epiphysis and diaphysis, are linked by hyaline cartilage which eventually ossifies. *Secondary* cartilaginous joints (*symphyses*) are joined by compressible fibrocartilage and reinforced by a surrounding tough fibrous capsule: they are predominantly axial (e.g. symphysis pubis, intervertebral joints, manubriosternal joints).

If a moderate or wide range of movement is required, a space must exist between the bones forming a discontinuous *diarthrosis* or *synovial joint* (Fig. 1.2). In synovial joints the bone ends are covered by hyaline cartilage, a firm but mildly compressible tissue ideally suited to load transmission. In some cases additional fibrocartilage pads divide the articular cavity completely (*discs*) or partially (*menisci*). An encircling *capsule* attaches between the bones: its outer portion is fibrous, its inner lining forms the villous *synovial membrane*. The latter has both secretory and macrophage functions. It produces the viscous modified ultrafiltrate—*synovial fluid*—that fills the potential 'joint space', being important in lubrication and nutrition of cartilage. In many joints the synovium has multiple inward facing processes containing fat (*plicae*). *Ligaments* insert between the bones as thickened portions of capsule or as separate structures. The site of firm attachment of fibrous structures (tendon, ligament, capsule) into periosteum and bone is called the *enthesis*, a site frequently inflamed through mechanical trauma or by involvement by inflammatory disease (particularly seronegative spondarthropathies).

Bursae are important fluid-filled sacs which facilitate smooth movement between articulating structures. Their lining lacks a basement membrane and appears identical to synovium.

- **Subcutaneous bursae** (e.g. olecranon, prepatellar bursae) form only after birth in response to normal external friction.
- **Deep bursae** (e.g. subacromial bursa) usually form before birth in response to movement between muscles and bones, and may or may not communicate with adjacent joint cavities.
- **'Adventitious' bursae** (e.g. over 1st metatarsal head) form in response to abnormal shearing stresses and are not uniformly present.

Muscles acting over the joint move it through its normal range. Forceful movement in one direction is always controlled by relaxation of the antagonist muscles: the balanced action of muscles thus constrains as well as powers joint movement.

Tendons act as functional and anatomical bridges between muscle and bone. Muscle is unnecessary for the early differentiation of tendon, but without good muscle strength sustained development of tendon fails. Many tendons, particularly those with a wide range of motion, have sheaths resembling the capsule/synovium of joints to permit easy gliding movement and to allow action as a pulley across acutely angled joints, such as the ankle.

The range of movement and stability of individual synovial joints varies according to:

- the shape of the articular surfaces,
- capsular strength,
- ligaments,
- muscles acting across the joint,
- the presence of adjacent structures.

Descriptive classification, especially of diarthrodial joints, is often based on the type of movement undertaken by the joint (Fig. 1.3).

PRINCIPLES OF THE RHEUMATOLOGICAL EXAMINATION

The rheumatological examination is very much an exercise in applied anatomy, with utilisation of simple provocation or stress tests to elicit signs. It cannot be overemphasised that examination of the locomotor system should form an integral part of the full general medical examination. Many rheumatic diseases have manifestations in other systems and, conversely, many 'general medical' conditions (particularly endocrine, metabolic and neoplastic) have locomotor manifestations. In this introductory section, only locomotor history and examination will be considered: an accompanying full systems enquiry and examination is assumed, and aspects relating only to key target sites of extralocomotor involvement will be emphasised.

Terminology

The following brief glossary relates to terms commonly used to describe the site and nature of locomotor problems:

Arthralgia. Pain arising from within joints (not necessarily with obvious abnormality).
Arthritis/Arthropathy. Objective joint abnormality.
Bursitis. Inflammation of a bursa.
Enthesopathy. Inflammation/abnormality of an enthesis.
Monoarthritis. Arthropathy of one joint only.
Myopathy. Disease/abnormality of muscle.
Myositis. Inflammatory disease of muscle.
Oligoarthritis/pauci-articular disease. Arthritis affecting two to four joints (or small joint groups, e.g. 'wrist').
Polyarthritis. Arthritis affecting more than four joints (or groups).
Synovitis. Clinically apparent synovial joint inflammation.
Tenosynovitis. Tendon sheath inflammation.
Tendinitis. Inflammation of tendon.
Tendonosis. Tendon degeneration.

Symptoms

Locomotor symptoms requiring clear delineation in the history are summarised in Table 1.1. It is important to ascertain:

- the site and distribution of involvement,
- chronological onset,
- preceding provoking factors,
- factors which worsen or improve symptoms,
- symptom response to health interventions.

Pain

Pain is the usual and most important symptom for which the patient seeks relief. The examiner must be in no doubt as to where the patient is experiencing pain. Patient vocabulary alone (e.g. 'shoulder', 'hip') may be misleading and the patient should be asked to point to and delineate on his or her body the area over which pain is felt and the site of maximum intensity.

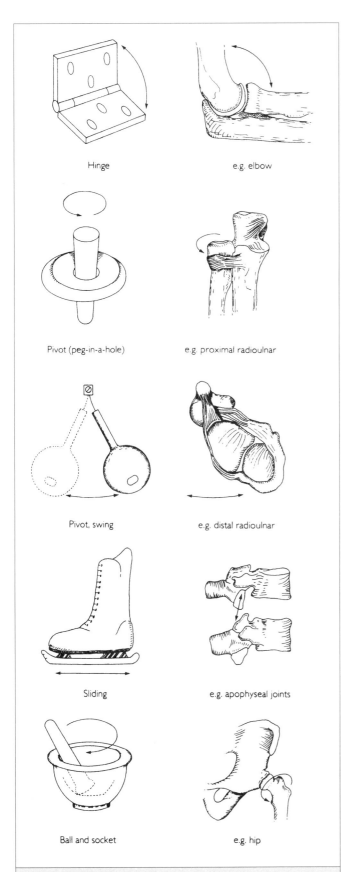

Fig. 1.3 Classification according to joint movement.

Hinge — e.g. elbow
Pivot (peg-in-a-hole) — e.g. proximal radioulnar
Pivot, swing — e.g. distal radioulnar
Sliding — e.g. apophyseal joints
Ball and socket — e.g. hip

Table 1.1. Important locomotor symptoms

- Pain:
    - site
    - radiation
    - quality
    - in usage
    - at rest
    - at night
- Stiffness:
    - morning
    - inactivity
- Swelling/deformity
- Disability
    - handicap
- Systemic illness
- Sleep disturbance/affect

Articular or periarticular pain may radiate widely and present distant from the originating structure (Fig. 1.4). Such pain felt elsewhere than at its origin is termed *referred*. Referred pain is an error in perception at the sensory cortex level, reflecting shared innervation from structures derived from the same embryonic segment (which divides into dermatome, myotome, sclerotome). Sensory (including painful) stimuli reaching cortical cells will most commonly originate from a certain area of skin: when the same cells receive for the first time a painful stimulus from a more deep-seated structure (myotomal or sclerotomal origin) they interpret the signal on past experience and 'feel' the pain in the area of skin (dermatome) connected with those particular cortical

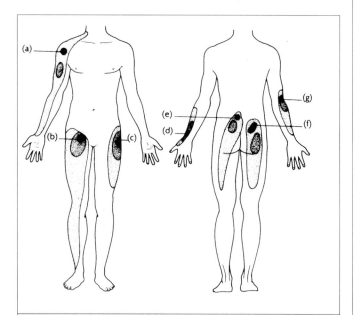

Fig. 1.4 Examples of pain radiation: (a) glenohumeral joint/rotator cuff, (b) hip joint, (c) trochanteric bursitis, (d) de Quervain's tenosynovitis, (e) lumbar facet joint syndrome, (f) sacroiliac joint, (g) tennis elbow syndrome. ■, origin of pain; ▨ , site of maximum pain; ☐ where pain is felt.

cells. An important difference, however, is that the pain is felt deeply rather than in the skin itself. Certain points are relevant to such referred pain:

- Pain radiates segmentally without crossing the midline.
- The extent of the relevant dermatome governs the distance pain may radiate. Extensive referral only occurs where elongated segments exist (i.e. limbs).
- The dermatome often extends more distally than the myotome, so pain is usually referred predominantly in a distal direction. The more distal the originating structure the more accurate the pain localisation is likely to be.
- Dermatomes are extremely variable between individuals—consequently, the precise pattern and area of pain referral may vary between individuals with the same originating musculoskeletal problem.
- In general, the more superficial a soft-tissue structure the more precise its localising ability. Pain is apt to be referred from capsule, ligament, muscle and bursa in an indistinguishable manner. Pain from bone and periosteum, however, hardly radiates at all and this discrepancy between soft and hard structures is unexplained.

Detailed questioning on the descriptive *quality* of pain is generally unhelpful. Exceptions, however, include (1) sharp shooting pain that travels a distance, characteristic of root entrapment, and (2) extreme pain ('worst experienced'), which is typical of crystal synovitis. Although topographical localisation of sensation is at the sensory cortex level, the fact that it is painful and the degree of pain experienced is determined by cells in the supraorbital region of the frontal lobes. Such localisation explains why the patient's emotional state has such a profound influence over pain 'severity'. The temporal lobes retain the memory of pain and it is the duration rather than the severity which principally determines recollection.

Factors which exacerbate or ameliorate the pain should obviously be sought. It is convenient to consider locomotor pain in terms of *usage*, *rest* and *night* pain. Pain confined to *usage* suggests a mechanical problem, particularly if it worsens during use and quickly improves on resting. *Rest pain* and pain worse at the beginning rather than end of usage implies a pronounced inflammatory component. *Night pain* is a distressing symptom that often carries a poor prognosis: it predominantly associates with marked intraosseous hypertension and may therefore denote serious problems such as avascular necrosis or subchondral bone collapse adjacent to a severely arthritic joint. Persistent day and night pain is particularly worrying, and such *bony pain* is characteristic of neoplastic invasion.

Stiffness

Stiffness is a sensation of tightness that can usually 'wear off'. In simplistic terms it can be thought of as fluid accumulation that distends the limiting boundary of the inflamed tissue (e.g. joint capsule, tenosynovium, bursa). It is most marked on (1) first arising in the morning (following relative inactivity during sleep), and (2) following inactivity or rest of the inflamed region. As the region resumes the movement of normal usage, fluid clearance from the inflamed structure is encouraged and stiffness 'wears off'. Duration and severity of *early morning* and *inactivity stiffness* are therefore important indicators of the degree of local inflammation.

Swelling/deformity

Patients themselves may notice swelling (which could be soft tissue, fluid or bone), discoloration or an abnormal contour or alignment of a locomotor structure. Strictly speaking, 'deformity' is anything out of the ordinary; the term is usually reserved, however, for a malalignment or subluxation/dislocation (the last two terms, rather than deformity, are preferable during discussions with the patient).

Disability and handicap

Disability is present when a tissue, organ or system is unable to perform its function adequately. Such disability may lead to *handicap* if it interferes with daily activities or social/occupational performance. Marked disability need not necessarily cause handicap (e.g. an above-knee amputee may not be disadvantaged in a sedentary job); similarly, minor disability may produce major handicap (e.g. a bunion in a professional athlete). The two must therefore be assessed separately, the history being particularly important in determining handicap.

Systemic illness

Inflammatory locomotor disease, particularly with multisystem involvement, may trigger a marked acute phase response and lead to symptoms of systemic upset. Patients may notice low-grade fevers (particularly at night), weight

loss, fatiguability, lethargy, and irritability. Often the patient volunteers no specific complaints but just feels generally 'ill' ('malaise'). In the elderly, in particular, florid inflammation (e.g. acute gout or pseudogout) may cause toxic confusion.

Sleep disturbance/affect

There may be several reasons for poor sleep in patients with locomotor disease:

- Any chronic painful condition may interfere with sleep (such interruption may play a part in the fibromyalgia syndrome).
- Triggering of the acute phase response may affect normal sleep patterns.
- Severe arthropathy (particularly hip and knee) may compromise sexual function, and contribute to marital/social disharmony.
- Latent anxiety and depression is not uncommon in patients with severe arthropathy, perhaps resulting from reasonable concern about deformity, function and morbidity.
- Some drugs used for pain relief (e.g. indomethacin) may produce central nervous system side-effects with alteration in sleep and mood.

Features of masked or overt depression (e.g. psychomotor retardation, constipation, weepiness, no thoughts of the future) should specifically be sought, particularly in those with severe locomotor problems. Poor sleep pattern is also a feature of fibromyalgia.

Signs

The principal headings for signs to be sought at any region are shown in Table 1.2. The order of examination applicable to most regions is:

1. inspection at rest,
2. inspection during movement,
3. palpation.

Attitude

Observation of the patient from the first contact is important, for example on walking into the examination room, and the way in which the patient positions an affected

Table 1.2. Important locomotor signs

- Attitude
- Deformity (correctable?)
- Skin changes
- Swelling:
  site
  fluid
  soft tissue
  bone
- Muscle wasting
- Tenderness:
  diffuse, point
  joint line
- Movement:
  range
  pain
- Crepitus
- Increased warmth
- Muscle strength
- Stability
- Function

region or limb may provide important clues to the underlying problem. Any inflamed joint with synovitis has intra-articular hypertension and is most comfortable in the position that minimises pressure increase. The position of maximum comfort is mainly determined by the capsule and the ligamentous arrangement: the position is that of greatest laxity which allows maximum intracapsular capacity ('loose-pack' position). In general, this is a position of mild–mid flexion (i.e. the fetal position). For example, a patient with glenohumeral synovitis (Fig. 1.5) is most comfortable if the arm is held in adduction and internal rotation (as if in a sling): equally, the earliest affected and most uncomfortable movements are the opposite of these, namely abduction and external rotation, since these maximally increase intra-articular pressure ('close-pack' position). The attitude and pattern of restricted movement may thus suggest the diagnosis.

Deformity

Although deformities may readily be observed at rest, many will become more apparent on weight bearing or usage. It should be determined whether the deformity is *correctable* (usually implying soft-tissue factors in causation) or *non-correctable* (more commonly capsular restriction, joint damage). Consider whether deformity at one site is secondary to deformity at a more proximal joint (e.g. knee flexion resulting from fixed flexion deformity of ipsilateral hip). Many conditions associate with characteristic deformities (e.g. at the knee, Fig. 1.6), but no deformity is pathognomonic of any one disease. Shorthand terms are often used for combined deformities (e.g. 'swan neck' deformity for hyperextension at the proximal and hyperflexion at the distal interphalangeal joints of the same finger).

Skin changes

Overlying traumatic/surgical scars or skin disease (e.g. psoriasis) may be important clues to causation. *Erythema* (commonly followed by desquamation) is an important sign that reflects periarticular inflammation. Although this may occur in several conditions (Table 1.3), a red joint (or bursa) should always raise suspicion of sepsis or crystals.

Fig. 1.5 Typical attitude of patient with glenohumeral synovitis.

Fig. 1.6 Principal knee deformities. (a) *Varus*: typical of osteoarthritis (a focal condition maximally affecting the medial compartment). (b) *Valgus*: typical of pancompartment inflammatory conditions, e.g. rheumatoid, psoriatic, pyrophosphate arthropathy. (c) *Recurvatum*: common in generalised hypermobility. (d) *Posterior tibial subluxation*: characteristic of arthritis occurring during growth, e.g. haemophilia. (e) *Fixed flexion*: common in various arthropathies.

Table 1.3. Causes of erythema overlying joints

MAJOR
Sepsis
Crystals (gout, pseudogout, calcific periarthritis)

MINOR
Palindromic rheumatism
Acute Reiter's syndrome, reactive arthropathy
Erythema nodosum
Early Heberden's and Bouchard's nodes
Rheumatic fever

Erythema implies associated periarticular inflammation

Warmth

This is one of the cardinal signs of inflammation and should be sought over bursae, tendon sheaths, entheses and joints (non-axial joints that are not deep in soft tissues are readily accessible for temperature assessment). The back of the hand is a sensitive thermometer for comparing skin temperature above, over and below an inflamed structure.

Swelling

This may be due to *fluid, soft tissue* or *bone*. Fluid within a joint collects initially and maximally at sites of least resistance within the capsular confines, producing a characteristic swelling at individual joint sites, for example:

- *A knee effusion* initially fills in the medial dimple at the side of the patella and subsequently the suprapatellar pouch, giving a horseshoe swelling above and to either side of the patella (Fig. 1.7).
- *Interphalangeal joint synovitis* is initially apparent as posterolateral swelling between the extensor tendon and lateral collateral ligaments (Fig. 1.8).
- *Glenohumeral effusion* initially fills the triangular depression between clavicle and deltoid in front of pectoralis.

For fluid within an anatomically confined space several signs may be elicited. A small fluid volume may produce a *bulge sign* if it is gently massaged from one side of the space to the other (readily demonstrable at the knee by flicking fluid from the medial dimple to the lateral aspect of the patella and back again; Fig. 1.9). A larger volume abolishes the bulge sign but permits elucidation of a *balloon sign* where pressure exerted at one point of the swelling is felt as 'ballooning' at other parts of the swelling (Fig. 1.10). This is the

Fig. 1.7 Appearance of knee effusion/synovial swelling: above and to either side of the patella.

Fig. 1.8 Appearance of swelling (posterolateral) caused by interphalangeal synovitis.

most specific sign for fluid in joints or bursae. *Capsular swelling* is the most specific sign of synovitis: swelling is delineated by the capsular confines and becomes firmer as the joint moves towards the extremes of movement (palpate during passive movement).

Fig. 1.9 The 'bulge' sign demonstrated at the knee. Fluid can be flicked from medial to lateral aspects ('dimples'). The other hand prevents movement from patella displacement.

Fig. 1.10 The 'balloon' sign demonstrated at the knee. With one hand pressing over the suprapatellar pouch, posterior pressure on the patella causes outward expansion of the other examining hand due to fluid confinement within the joint.

Tenderness

Precise localisation of tenderness is perhaps the most useful sign in determining the cause of the patient's problem.

Joint-line/capsular tenderness is localised to the joint boundary and signifies arthropathy or capsular disease if present around the whole joint margin. Localised, rather than generalised, joint-line tenderness may reflect problems with an intracapsular structure (e.g. anterior medial tibiofemoral compartment tenderness at the knee is common with medial meniscal tears).

Periarticular point tenderness away from the joint line usually signifies bursitis or enthesopathy.

Movement

The range of both *active* and *passive* movement can readily be assessed with comparison of one side with the other. Synovitis usually reduces most or all joint movements (although some are affected initially and maximally, e.g. external rotation and abduction at the glenohumeral joint). Each joint has a characteristic pattern of such 'proportional' limitation ('*capsular pattern*'), governed largely by the capsular and ligamentous arrangement that determines intracapsular pressure changes on movement. Tenosynovitis and periarticular lesions more commonly affect movement in one plane only (i.e. the plane of movement of the involved structure). Such a '*non-capsular*' pattern of restriction may also result from an internal derangement (only certain joints such as the knee and elbow are affected in this way). Synovitis and arthropathy usually result in similar reduction of both active and passive movement: passive movement far greater than active movement suggests a muscle/tendon/motor problem.

The pattern of pain elicited by movement is of great diagnostic significance. Pain absent or minimal in the mid-range position but increasing progressively towards the extremes of restricted movement is *stress pain* (Fig. 1.11). *Universal stress pain* (i.e. in most/all directions) is the most sensitive sign of synovitis (Table 1.4). *Selective stress pain* (i.e. in one plane of movement only) is characteristic of a localised lesion in or around a joint. Pain uniformly present throughout a range of movement usually reflects mechanical rather than inflammatory problems.

Ranges of joint movement are age-, sex- and race-dependent, and are difficult to quantify with any accuracy (other than by radiographic techniques). Direct comparison of one side with the other may be helpful in demonstrating unilateral reduction or increase. Attempts to measure degrees of movement (by a variety of instruments) are inaccurate, have poor reproducibility and are not recommended.

A principle used at several sites for demonstrating muscle tendon or enthesis problems is *resisted active (isometric) movement* (Fig. 1.12). The patient is asked to push against the

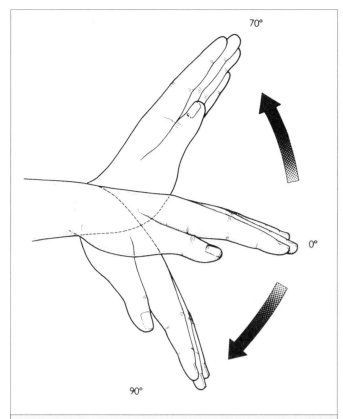

Fig. 1.11 'Stress pain' at the wrist: no discomfort in mild flexion, but progressive pain towards the extremes of restricted flexion and extension.

Table 1.4. Characteristic findings in an inflamed joint (synovitis), tenosynovitis and a damaged joint

SYNOVITIS
Most comfortable in neutral position
Decreased movement *all* planes
Stress pain *all* directions
Capsular swelling/effusion
Joint-line/capsular tenderness
Warmth
± Fine crepitus
Capsular swelling = most specific sign
Stress pain = most sensitive sign

TENOSYNOVITIS
Joint positioned to decrease tension on tendon
Decreased movement in plane of tendon
Selective stress pain
Linear swelling
Localised (linear) tenderness
± Fine crepitus
± Triggering

JOINT DAMAGE
Abnormal shape
Coarse crepitus
Decreased movement
± Ligamentous stress pain/instability
± Synovitis

Fig. 1.12 Restricted active movement and stress tests. (a) Attempted external rotation at the shoulder causing upper arm pain in infraspinatus/teres minor rotator cuff lesion. (b) Resisted wrist extension reproducing lateral epicondyle pain in tennis elbow. (c) Finkelstein's test: passive ulnar flexion with the thumb held stretches abductor pollicis longus and extensor pollicis brevis to reproduce pain of de Quervain's tenosynovitis.

examiner's restraining hand, to contract the muscle of interest without moving adjacent joints (to minimise the chance of joint or surrounding inert tissue movement, the joint is placed in a neutral or resting position). If the patient's pain is reproduced by this manoeuvre (and no joint or surrounding inert tissue has moved) it is likely that the pain arises from the muscle, tendon or tendon insertion related to that movement. For example, resisted adduction at the hip may reproduce medial groin pain in adductor tendonitis, resisted glenohumeral abduction may produce upper arm pain with supraspinatus muscle or tendon lesions and resisted active wrist extension may produce pain at the lateral epicondyle in tennis elbow. Similarly, *passive stress tests* may be applied in an attempt to reproduce the patient's pain by stretching the responsible ligament or tendon (e.g. Finkelstein's test for de Quervain's tenosynovitis, where passive stretch of abductor pollicis longus and extensor pollicis brevis reproduces pain).

Crepitus

Crepitus is palpable crunching present throughout the range of movement of the involved structure. *Fine crepitus* may be audible by stethoscope and is not transmitted through bone adjacent to the involved structure; it may accompany inflammation of tendon sheath, bursa or synovium. *Coarse crepitus* may be audible at a distance and is often palpable through adjacent bone: it usually reflects cartilage or bone damage. Other locomotor noises include *ligamentous snaps* (usually single, loud and painless: commonly heard around the greater trochanter region as 'clicking hips'), *cracking* by joint distraction (common at finger joints and caused by formation of an intra-articular gas bubble subsequent to the negative pressure generated: such painless and inconsequential 'cracking' cannot be repeated until the bubble has resorbed) and a variety of reproducible *clonking* noises at irregular surfaces (e.g. moving the scapula over the thoracic wall).

Muscle

Muscle wasting is a common but difficult sign, particularly in women and older patients in whom muscle contour is normally less striking. Synovitis will quickly produce reflex inhibition of muscles acting across the joint by local spinal reflex: wasting of muscle can occur very quickly (e.g. within 2–3 days in septic arthritis). Severe arthropathy commonly produces widespread wasting of muscles around the joint: localised wasting is more characteristic of a mechanical tendon/muscle problem or peripheral nerve damage. Power is more important than bulk and should be tested, either by formal testing using MRC grades 0–5 (Table 1.5: appropriate, for example, for proximal girdle and neck muscle weakness

Table 1.5.   Muscle power grading (Medical Research Council scale)

Grade	Muscle power
0	No visible contraction
1	Visible or palpable contraction without motion
2	Motion only with gravity eliminated
3	Motion against gravity
4	Motion against gravity and an applied load
5	Normal, i.e. against a significant load

in polymyositis) or by assessment of functional capabilities (suitable, for example, for weakness of small hand muscles in polyarticular rheumatoid).

Stability

Localised ligamentous or capsular instability may result from traumatic or inflammatory lesions: direct comparison with the other side (and with other joints) should always be made in case this represents part of generalised hypermobility. Inflammatory joint disease (particularly rheumatoid) may produce instability via cartilage loss and capsular inflammation, as well as by ligamentous rupture.

Function

Function for each joint region is assessed by observation during normal usage (e.g. rising from chair and walking, for assessing hips, knees and feet; power grip and fine precision pinch for assessing the hand). *Activities of daily living* (e.g. dressing, brushing teeth, turning handles, going to the toilet unaided, cooking) are of principal relevance to the patient, and screening questions or observations of such movements ('ADL') are invaluable in assessment. Handicap is mainly determined by questioning in respect of work and social activities. A number of tested and validated questionnaires/scoring systems are available for *functional* and *quality of life assessments*. The latter particularly depends on physical, psychological and emotional factors, which are highly specific to the patient rather than to the condition.

Two generalised conditions are easily missed unless specifically considered:

Generalised hypermobility. Approximately 10% of people fall within the lax end of a normal spectrum of joint mobility. Although normal, such hypermobility may contribute to locomotor problems (e.g. enthesopathy, dislocation). Within this 10% are also the small number of individuals with disease-related hypermobility (e.g. Marfan's syndrome, Ehlers–Danlos syndrome, acromegaly). Generalised hypermobility can be screened for using a modified Beighton score (Table 1.6).

Fibromyalgia (non-restorative sleep disorder). This common syndrome is characterised by:

- poor sleep pattern (waking unrefreshed),
- fatiguability, lethargy,
- irritability, weepiness,
- multiple regional pain problems (predominantly axial, often 'all over'), usually unresponsive to analgesics,
- hypersensitivity of normal tender sites (Fig. 1.13),
- frequent accompanying 'tension' headaches and irritable bowel syndrome.

Fibromyalgia predominates in women and increases in prevalence with age. It is suggested by the features in the history and confirmed principally by the finding of hypertender sites (with no hyperalgesia at other, control sites such as the forehead and distal forearm) and elimination of other causes of widespread aches and pains (e.g. hyperparathyroidism, hypothyroidism, lupus, etc.). Unless specifically considered it is easily missed.

Recording of locomotor signs

Although it is feasible to record physical findings in note form, annotation around skeleton charts or homunculi (Fig.

Table 1.6. Generalised hypermobility defined using a Carter and Wilkinson score (modified by Beighton)

Extend little finger > 90° (1 point each)
Bring back thumb parallel to/touching forearm (1 point each)
Extend elbow > 10° (1 point each)
Extend knee > 10° (1 point each)
Touch floor with flat of hands, legs straight (1 point)
Maximum score = 9 (6+ = hypermobile)

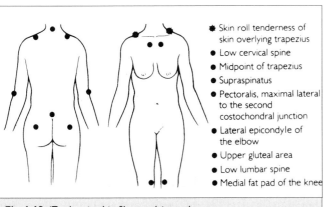

* Skin roll tenderness of skin overlying trapezius
• Low cervical spine
• Midpoint of trapezius
• Supraspinatus
• Pectoralis, maximal lateral to the second costochondral junction
• Lateral epicondyle of the elbow
• Upper gluteal area
• Low lumbar spine
• Medial fat pad of the knee

Fig. 1.13 'Tender sites' in fibromyalgia syndrome.

1.14) is strongly recommended. Such a visual method of recording greatly aids pattern recognition.

Aspects of the general examination

In the context of a complete systems examination particular emphasis may be given to skin (including scalp, umbilicus and natal cleft for occult psoriasis), nails, mucous membranes and eyes. It cannot be overemphasised, however, that a full medical history and examination should be undertaken.

Nodules are a feature of particular relevance to locomotor disease (Table 1.7). Whatever the cause, they are usually most prominent over extensor surfaces with poor soft-tissue covering (e.g. back of hand, elbow, posterior heel, sacrum).

Table 1.7. Causes of nodules and arthropathy

COMMON
Rheumatoid arthritis
Gout (= 'tophi')
Hyperlipidaemia (= 'xanthomata')

RARE
Systemic lupus erythematosus (small nodules)
Rheumatic fever
Polyarteritis nodosa
Multicentric reticulohistiocytosis
Sarcoidosis

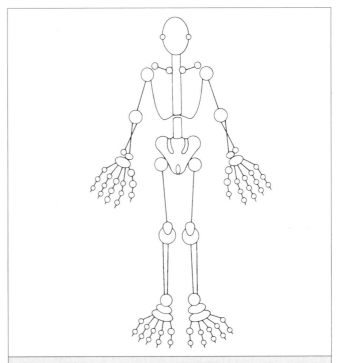

Fig. 1.14 'Homunculus' for annotated recording of locomotor signs.

Nail changes of interest include clubbing (most causes of clubbing have locomotor associations, but hypertrophic pulmonary osteoarthropathy and fibrosing alveolitis are particularly relevant), 'thimble pitting', onycholysis and nail dystrophy (psoriatic arthropathy, chronic Reiter's syndrome) and splinter haemorrhages (small vessel vasculitis). Rheumatoid arthritis is the commonest pathological cause of *palmar erythema* (more so than cirrhosis and thyrotoxicosis; pregnancy is a common physiological cause).

Mucous membrane lesions may be asymptomatic (Reiter's/reactive arthropathy) or symptomatic (usual in lupus, vasculitides, Behçet's syndrome), and inspection of orogenital and nasal mucosae for ulcers and telangiectasia is warranted. Absence of saliva either side of the frenulum suggests sicca syndrome (patients often complain of dry mouth, particularly in the morning, and difficulty swallowing certain foods: dry eyes are more commonly asymptomatic).

Eye changes (Table 1.8) include episcleritis and scleritis (rheumatoid arthritis, vasculitides, polychondritis), iritis (ankylosing spondylitis, chronic Reiter's syndrome), iridocyclitis (pauciarticular juvenile chronic arthritis), and conjunctivitis (acute Reiter's syndrome, sicca syndrome). A Schirmer tear test is a simple screen for sicca syndrome; although it may produce false positives and negatives, it may readily be performed without special equipment (Fig. 1.15). Confirmation of sicca syndrome is by rose bengal

Table 1.8. Important causes of a red eye

CONJUNCTIVITIS
Itchiness, irritation
Diffusely red due to engorged vessel network
Redness extends over bulbar surface of eyelids
Vessels can be moved over surface
Mucopurulent discharge common ('sticky eye')

EPISCLERITIS
Usually asymptomatic
Diffuse or localised ('nodular' episcleritis)
Bright red flush, individual vessels often visible
Vessels cannot be moved over eyeball
Vessels constrict to local adrenaline drops (1:1000)

SCLERITIS
Usually painful, often severe
Deep red/purple colour, vessels indistinct
Deep vessels do not constrict with adrenaline drops
Often accompanied by episcleritis
Localised ('nodular') scleritis causes elevated lesion due to oedema
Diffuse scleritis causes less pain but may involve cornea, causing keratitis and keratolysis ('corneal melt')
Healed scleritis may leave sclera more transparent and permit the dark underlying choroid to be seen

ACUTE IRITIS
Severe, throbbing pain
Blurring of vision, photophobia, lacrimation
Usually involves only one eye at a time: light in other eye will exacerbate pain as iris constricts
Small vessels of limbus are engorged ('ciliary flush')
Small spastic pupil, may be irregular (due to posterior adhesions or synechiae)
Clouding of aqueous ± (anterior chamber pus collection inferiorly ('hypopyon')

staining and slit-lamp examination (histological evidence is most commonly sought by lip biopsy to show minor salivary gland changes).

Assimilation of findings

Following the history and examination it is often helpful to organise findings under the titles in Table 1.9. Making a diagnosis rarely presents problems once the clinically derived information is collected and considered. Problems and misdiagnosis most commonly arise if an inadequate or inaccurate history and examination have failed to elicit the correct information in the first instance.

Consideration just of age and gender will narrow diagnostic possibilities considerably. Occasionally, genetic factors (race, family history) may suggest or support a particular diagnosis, though a positive history (which may of course be inaccurate in terms of precise diagnosis in family members) is as often as misleading as it is helpful, and most store should be placed on the individual patient findings. For arthropathy in a patient of a certain age and sex the temporal

Distance of wetness from lid is measured after 3 minutes

Blotting paper strip

Fig. 1.15 Schirmer tear test.

Table 1.9.   Principal considerations when organising findings

Patient characteristics
- Age
- Gender
- Family history/race
- Occupation/recreations

Onset, chronology of symptoms
- Acute/insidious
- Chronic
- Periodic/relapsing

?Extra-articular features

Periarticular ('soft-tissue') problem
- Single regional
  ?trauma/strain/overusage
- Multiple regional
  ?fibromyalgia
  ?multisystem disease

Articular problem
- Number of joints involved
  monoarticular
  oligo-/pauciarticular
  polyarticular
- Distribution
  small joints/large joints
  upper limb, lower limb, axial
  symmetrical/asymmetrical
- Inflammatory component

presentation (acute, chronic or relapsing), number of joints involved, distribution, and degree of inflammatory component (assessed from both symptoms and signs) will usually suggest the most likely diagnosis, with a few alternatives. The presence of particular extra-articular features may narrow possibilities further. Investigations, if required, can then be highly selected, and a rheumatological 'screen' with multiple investigations should never be necessary. It should be remembered, however, that apparently mundane and localised lesions (e.g. Achilles tendinitis) may be the presenting feature of a more widespread or multisystem condition.

Only an adequate history and examination will permit correct diagnosis and an appropriate management plan.

2

The minimum rheumatological examination

In terms of physical examination the locomotor system is extensive and complex. An exhaustive history and examination for all conceivable rheumatological abnormalities in every patient would not only be very time-consuming but also inefficient and unnecessary. As with the neurological examination (and to a lesser extent other systems examination), a brief screening procedure to pick up problems in certain regions is more appropriate. If an abnormality is detected, more detailed examination of the affected region(s) (as described in subsequent chapters) can then be undertaken.

A screening procedure represents a compromise between brevity and reasonable sensitivity for detecting abnormality. Every physician must develop his or her own personal variation of the 'minimum survey' for the locomotor just as for other systems, and the procedure described in this section is offered as a guide rather than didactic doctrine. Such a survey, however, is reasonable to include as a 'minimal statement' within the systems enquiry and examination screen that comprises the routine medical clerking. Furthermore, such a survey should form a component of the basic examination that lies within the scope of all practising doctors and is performed so routinely as to become 'reflex' in nature. Certain aspects of the screen (e.g. gait) might be undertaken during screening of other systems and, in the context of a full examination, takes only an extra minute or so to perform. The following screen has been validated in a general medical setting and shown to be sensitive at detecting locomotor abnormality and functional impairment.

SCREENING HISTORY

Pain and stiffness are the two most common symptoms relating to locomotor abnormality, and impairment of function is the most important common consequence. The following are therefore reasonable screening questions for rheumatological disease:

Have you any pain or stiffness in your muscles, joints or back?
Can you dress yourself completely without any difficulty?
Can you walk up and down stairs without any difficulty?

Dressing is a daily event and one with which the patient will readily identify in terms of problems. Ability to dress completely (including shoes and socks) is a sensitive functional test of most upper and lower limb joints, and if the patient has no pain or difficulty performing this task then significant or widespread locomotor disease is unlikely. If the patient can ascend and descend stairs without pain or difficulty then most lower limb muscles and joints (large and small) are functioning well: walking on the flat is also unlikely to present problems (up and down stairs is a better test of hip and knee, particularly patellofemoral, problems than walking on the flat). If none of these questions pick up a problem then further questioning is unlikely to do so. If a problem is detected, more detailed questioning should obviously be undertaken.

SCREENING EXAMINATION

The main emphasis is on inspection at rest and inspection during selected movements which are affected early by joint disease. Brief palpation and stress tests of target joint sites (e.g. metacarpophalangeal joints—MCPJs, metatarsophalangeal joints—MTPJs, knees) complete the screen.

If a joint is normal it should:

1. *Look normal.* With advancing age the surface contours of a joint become more visible, and muscle bulk diminishes, without necessarily having pathological significance.
2. *Assume a normal resting position.* Each joint has a characteristic resting position. Abnormal positioning of a normal joint may result from poor posture, neurological abnormality, or psychogenic disorder with feigning of

disease. Postural abnormalities should disappear once the patient is asked to adopt the normal position and undertake normal movements.

3. *Move smoothly through its range of movement.* Articular or periarticular lesions often result in a jerky, guarded movement, and the patient may utilise trick manoeuvres to minimise any functional problem.

The order of screening is of little consequence. Each practitioner develops his or her own order and, with practice, inspection, palpation and stress tests of a region can often be undertaken at the same time. Description of the patient assessment is conveniently considered during three activities: during walking, while standing and while lying on a couch. Observation of the patient getting undressed is a further useful screen to detect functional problems in upper and lower limb joints (though some physicians prefer to spare the patient any embarrassment this may cause).

Inspection of the walking patient

With the patient barefoot and undressed to his or her underwear, observe the patient's gait over a minimum of several yards as he or she walks forwards, turns and walks back again. Carefully inspect movements of the arms, pelvis, hips, knees, hindfoot, midfoot and forefoot in turn. Normal gait (Fig. 2.1) is characterised by:

- easy, flowing movement of each arm linked with coordinated movement of the opposite leg;
- symmetrical movement of the pelvis, smoothly rotating forward with the advancing leg;

- flexion of the hip at heel-strike, extension at toe-off;
- knee extension at heel-strike, flexion during swing;
- normal heel-strike, foot pronation in mid-stance, heel rise before push-off, and ankle dorsiflexion during swing;
- smooth turning ability.

As the patient walks and turns look particularly for an *antalgic gait*; where, pain or deformity causes the patient to hurry off one leg and to spend most of the gait cycle on the other. The type of antalgic gait may suggest the region that is abnormal. For example:

Low back problem. Decreased rotation of the pelvis with the advancing leg leads to a shortened step and caution when turning.

Hip problem. The body 'bobs' over the painful side: fixed flexion accentuates lumbar lordosis and exaggerates buttock prominence.

Knee problem. Synovitis/deformity may prevent full extension during swing and soften heel-strike. If the knee is ankylosed or held stiffly, the body pivots around the leg during stance phase and the leg is swung forward by circumduction.

Hindfoot problem. If movement through the ankle is reduced, the leg may be externally rotated and slightly abducted. With heel pain, heel-strike may be replaced by 'foot-strike': the heel is kept off the floor and the knee does not fully extend. With Achilles tendon problems, push-off is avoided.

Fig. 2.1 Main phases of gait (nearest leg): (a) heel-strike; (b) loading/stance; (c) toe-off; (d) swing.

Midfoot problem. The foot is held inverted (supinated) and push-off is from the lateral side.

Forefoot problem. To prevent weight-bearing on the forefoot the heel does not rise in late stance, and there is no push-off. The knee, hip and trunk flex to maintain forward motion, and swing phase on the normal side is shortened, resulting in forward 'bobbing' during late stance on the painful side. Involvement of both forefeet combines to give a forward leaning, short-stepped, shuffling gait.

Additional abnormalities include a *Trendelenburg gait* (the pelvis drops down on the opposite side during stance phase on the affected side—due to ineffective hip abduction), a *waddling gait* (i.e. a bilateral Trendelenburg gait), and *hysterical/psychogenic* gaits (often variable, exaggerated or bizarre, conforming to no easily recognised pattern).

If the observed gait is entirely normal, the patient is unlikely to have any major locomotor abnormality in the lower limbs or lumbar spine.

Inspection of the standing patient

Ask the patient to stand upright with arms outstretched by their sides.

1. Inspect from behind (Fig. 2.2), comparing one side with the other, looking particularly for:

- a straight spine (no scoliosis or rib-cage asymmetry);
- similar level of both iliac crests;
- normal muscle bulk/symmetry, especially around the shoulder and pelvic girdles, and the lumbar spine;
- popliteal swelling;
- swelling/asymmetry around the Achilles tendons;
- hindfoot deformity (valgus/varus).

While in this position apply pressure to the midpoint of each supraspinatus (Fig. 2.3), and undertake skinfold rolling of overlying skin (Fig. 2.4) looking for increased tenderness

Fig. 2.3 Applied pressure over midpoint of supraspinatus.

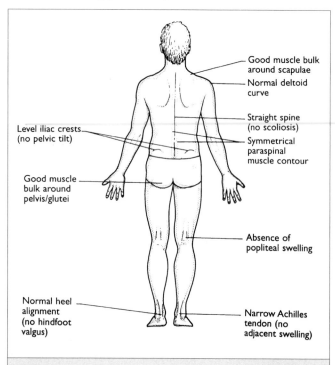

Good muscle bulk around scapulae

Normal deltoid curve

Level iliac crests (no pelvic tilt)

Straight spine (no scoliosis)

Symmetrical paraspinal muscle contour

Good muscle bulk around pelvis/glutei

Absence of popliteal swelling

Normal heel alignment (no hindfoot valgus)

Narrow Achilles tendon (no adjacent swelling)

Fig. 2.2 Inspection of the standing patient from behind—important items to check.

Fig. 2.4 Skinfold rolling (for fibromyalgia).

suggestive of fibromyalgia (these being two common sites of involvement).

2. Inspect from the side (Fig. 2.5), looking particularly for:

- loss of normal cervical and lumbar lordosis, and alteration of normal mild thoracic kyphosis,
- knee deformity (fixed flexion, genu recurvatum, posterior tibial subluxation).

While in this position, test lumbar spine and hip flexion by placing several fingers over the posterior spinous processes of the lower lumbar vertebrae and asking the patient to *bend forwards and touch his or her toes* as best as possible (Fig. 2.6). The thoracolumbar spine should form a smooth curve and the palpating fingers move apart if the lumbar spine is normal: a good range of movement implies normal hip flexion.

3. Inspect from in front (Fig. 2.7), comparing one side with the other. Look particularly for:

- swelling, abnormal position, skin change over each sternoclavicular and acromioclavicular joint site;
- equal shoulder height;

- muscle wasting/asymmetry, especially of deltoids and quadriceps;
- inability to fully extend elbows;
- deformity (particularly varus, valgus) of knee;

Fig. 2.6 Inspection/palpation of patient attempting to 'touch the toes'.

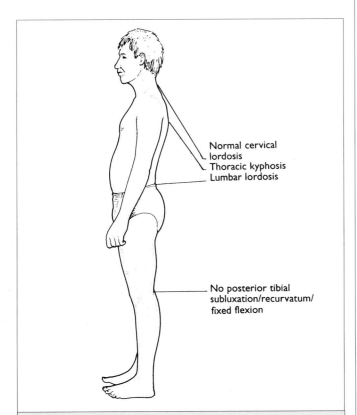

Fig. 2.5 Inspection of the standing patient from the side—important items to check.

Normal cervical lordosis
Thoracic kyphosis
Lumbar lordosis

No posterior tibial subluxation/recurvatum/fixed flexion

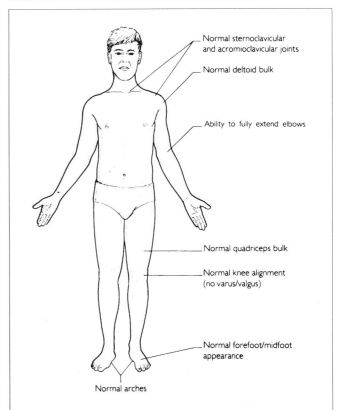

Fig. 2.7 Inspection of the standing patient from in front—important items to check.

Normal sternoclavicular and acromioclavicular joints

Normal deltoid bulk

Ability to fully extend elbows

Normal quadriceps bulk

Normal knee alignment (no varus/valgus)

Normal forefoot/midfoot appearance

Normal arches

- deformity (particularly of hallux, MTPJs) of forefoot and alteration of foot arches (flat feet).

While in this position ask the patient to:

1. *Laterally flex the neck* to each side (Fig. 2.8), looking for pain or restriction (lateral flexion is a sensitive test for cervical spine abnormality).
2. *Open the jaw wide and move it from side to side* (Fig. 2.9). It should open easily, without deviation to either side, sufficiently wide to accommodate three fingers vertically.
3. *Place both hands behind the head* with elbows right back (Fig. 2.10). External rotation and abduction are the earliest, most severely affected glenohumeral movements. This action also moves the acromioclavicular and sternoclavicular joints, and tests the supraspinatus, infraspinatus and teres minor.
4. *Place both hands out in front, palms down, fingers straight,* with elbows at 90° at the side (Fig. 2.11). Inspect for abnormalities (particularly swelling, deformity, attitude and skin changes) at the distal radioulnar joint, wrists, MCPJs and interphalangeal joints (IPJs). Look for the swelling of extensor tenosynovitis.
5. *Turn the hands over* (supination, Fig. 2.12, testing proximal and distal radioulnar joints). Inspect the palmar aspects, particularly for wasting, skin changes, flexor tenosynovitis swelling.
6. *Make a tight fist with each hand* (Fig. 2.13). Observe ability to curl fingers tightly into palms (power grip).

Fig. 2.9 'Open your mouth wide, and move it from side to side'.

Fig. 2.10 'Place your hands behind your head, elbows back'.

Fig. 2.8 'Place your ear on your left, then right shoulder'.

Fig. 2.11 Inspect dorsal aspects of the hands.

7. *Place the tip of each finger onto the tip of the thumb in turn* (Fig. 2.14). Observe dexterity for fine precision pinch.
8. *Squeeze across the 2nd to 5th metacarpals* (Fig. 2.15).

Fig. 2.12 Inspect palmar aspects of the hands.

Fig. 2.13 Observe a tight fist (power grip).

Fig. 2.14 Observe fine precision pinch.

Fig. 2.15 Metacarpal squeeze.

When asking the patient to undertake such specific actions it is often helpful for the examiner to do the same so that the patient can see exactly what is required (this speeds up the examination considerably).

Inspection/examination of the patient lying on a couch

Elderly patients particularly may find it uncomfortable to lie totally flat, and a sitting up position is adequate for screening manoeuvres. With the patient reclining comfortably:

1. *Flex the hip and knee while holding the knee* (Fig. 2.16). Ensure normal knee flexion and feel for crepitus. This again tests hip flexion.
2. *Passively internally rotate the hip* with the hip still flexed (Fig. 2.17). This is a sensitive test for hip disease. Repeat the last two procedures on the other side.

Fig. 2.16 Flexion of the hip and knee.

Fig. 2.17 Internal rotation of the flexed hip.

Fig. 2.18 Patellofemoral stress test and palpation for balloon sign.

Fig. 2.19 Metatarsal squeeze.

3. *Press down on the patella and palpate for a balloon sign in each knee* (Fig. 2.18). This tests the patellofemoral compartment and for synovitis in a joint commonly affected by all arthropathies.
4. *Squeeze all the metatarsals* (Fig. 2.19) to test the MTPJs.
5. *Inspect the soles for callosities.*

There are many other simple movements and tests that can be added to such a screen, although if findings for all of the above are normal it is very unlikely, in the face of a normal locomotor history screen, that significant abnormalities will be present. Other features of possible relevance to locomotor disease (e.g. nail changes, clubbing) will have been included in the screening of other systems.

3

Disease assessment indices and outcome measures

Measurement of disease activity and severity is necessary to assess patients' needs, monitor progress and evaluate the effects of interventions. Traditional measures of severity have concentrated on clinical or laboratory assessments. More recently it has been possible to measure other consequences of disease, including disability, psychological effects and overall health status. The World Health Organisation, in its publication, *The International Classification of Impairments, Disabilities and Handicaps*, has given guidance in considering these factors. Impairments refer to abnormalities of anatomical, physiological or psychological structure or function. It signifies that a pathological state has reached a stage of detectability. Examples include pain, weakness and stiffness and estimates of subjective 'wellbeing'. Disabilities are limitations in the performance of tasks in activities (such as walking and dressing). Handicaps refer to the disadvantages suffered because of ill health, and take into consideration the availability of help and resources, and the importance of different activities to the individual. Until recently the measurement of handicap in the rheumatic diseases has attracted little attention.

The relationships between impairments, disabilities and handicaps are important. Disease activity and progression is assessed using measures of impairment which are assumed to be fairly objective. Measuring disability is also well described. However, handicap may be the most important factor for the patient, because it can be reduced even when impairment and disability cannot, by, for example, modifying environment or social benefits.

In recent years there has been a growing interest in recording the patients' disease course in a standardised and reproducible way. Outcome measures must be valid and reliable whatever the setting but the relative importance of sensitivity to change and feasibility varies. Outcome measures may be divided into two broad categories, observer dependent or observer independent (self-rated). In clinical trials, sensitivity to change is important, whereas the choice of tests in the clinic depends on feasibility.

Bellamy (1993) has considered criteria that might be useful in selecting an existing assessment technique or in guiding the development of new techniques.

Major criteria

1. The measurement process must be ethical.
2. Reliability should be adequate for achieving measurement objectives.
3. Validity (content, criteria and construct) should be adequate for achieving measurement objectives.
4. Responsiveness must be adequate, i.e. the technique must be able to detect a clinically important, statistically significant change in the underlying variable.

Minor criteria

5. The technique should have been designed for a specific purpose.
6. The technique should have been validated in individuals or populations of patients having characteristics similar to future study populations.
7. The technique should have been adopted by other clinical investigators.
8. Performance should have been maintained in subsequent applications under similar study conditions.
9. The method of deriving scores, particularly in composite indices, should be both credible and comprehensible.
10. The feasibility of data collection and instrument application should not be constrained unduly by time or cost.

DISEASE ACTIVITY

In many rheumatic diseases, disease activity measures are attempts to quantify the inflammatory process and include the following aspects.

Pain

Pain is a subjective phenomenon, the perception of which is modulated by a variety of influences, and results in pain behaviours.

The alleviation of pain is one of the major goals of treatment of arthritis. Pain may be a consequence of either disease activity or disease damage, but the quantification of pain is part of disease assessment in most rheumatic diseases. It is usually assessed by using questionnaires. The response is then measured on a 10 cm visual analogue scale (VAS) or a five- point Likert-categorical scale. The McGill Pain Questionnaire (Melzak, 1975) is a popular longer questionnaire but has not proved superior to either VAS or Likert scales, and is more time-consuming.

A VAS may be used for pain intensity (least possible pain to worst possible pain) or pain relief (no relief of pain to complete relief of pain). Straight, horizontal and ungraded lines are the most sensitive. Categorical scales usually include either five (nil, slight, moderate, severe, agony) or four (none, mild, moderate, severe) assessments. Studies have shown that pain scales are a very sensitive measure in short- and medium-term drug trials and show reliability and sensitivity to change. There is less information as to their use over long periods of time; there are suggestions that it plateaus. Therefore pain may be more useful in measuring treatment in the short term, rather than monitoring disease progression.

When applying pain scales, it is important to specify the aspect of pain which is being assessed (e.g. walking, rest, night) and the time interval over which pain is being evaluated.

Morning stiffness and fatigue

Measurement of duration of morning stiffness (not severity) has been a popular measure in trials, whereas fatigue is only rarely mentioned. Neither measure is well standardised. However, stiffness may be less responsive than pain because up to 30% of rheumatoid patients do not experience stiffness at baseline in trials. It has been shown that stiffness is a poor discriminator between inflammatory and non-inflammatory joint disease, and duration of stiffness was also unable to discriminate between active and inactive rheumatoid arthritis.

Articular indices

The assessment of joint involvement is of prime importance in the evaluation of a patient's disease, both in clinical trials and in daily practice. There are a large number of different assessment methods. Most articular indices were developed for use in rheumatoid arthritis. They include a count of the number of swollen joints. Joint tenderness is an assessment of pain and both need to be assessed as there is only a fair correlation between them. The methods available vary in the number of joints assessed; joints may be 'weighted' according to size of the joint [the Thompson articular index (Thompson et al., 1988)]. The joint abnormality may be scored on a linear scale or recorded as abnormal or normal. A joint score is obtained when the abnormality is graded and the grades of all investigated joints summated. A joint count records the number of abnormal joints. Joint counts are more reproducible than joint scores, especially after standardisation of observers. They have been shown to correlate with current but not future disability.

The first articular index was introduced by Lansbury (1958) and measured tenderness or pain on movement in 84 joints. The American Rheumatism Association joint count is the standard articular index in use in North America. It uses a present/absent scale to record joint tenderness and/or pain on movement, and/or soft-tissue swelling in 68 joints. The Ritchie articular index is the most frequently used index in Europe (Ritchie et al., 1968); it assesses 53 joints for tenderness on a four-point scale and is really an objective measure of pain.

Doing a complete joint count is time-consuming and attempts have been made to simplify the instrument without losing validity. A case can be made, especially in routine practice, for changing to a 28-joint Fuchs index (Fuchs et al., 1989), which involves examining the metacarpophalangeal, proximal interphalangeal, shoulder, elbow, wrist and knee joints, and recording how many are tender and how many are swollen. This is a quicker assessment and has been well validated.

Articular indices have also been developed for other forms of arthritis. The Doyle index (Doyle et al., 1981) is an adaptation of the Ritchie index for use in osteoarthritis. The assessment of all joint areas in osteoarthritis may not always be appropriate as the disease is often present in only a few large joints.

Global assessments

Disease activity may be measured by assessing symptoms, signs, laboratory tests and imaging techniques. However, they may give confusing answers when some measures suggest disease improvement, and others deterioration. There has therefore been an attempt to pool several activity measures. The physician global assessment is the simplest form of composite index. A judgement of the patient's overall disease activity is made after assessing clinical and laboratory information. Global assessments predict future disability and are among the most sensitive to change in trials whilst retaining reliability. However, the questions asked in the assessment are not standardised. The scope of the assessment (all the ways your disease affects your general health), the time-frame (today, this last week) and response type all vary between studies.

An alternative is to use a pooled index consisting of a number of measures of disease activity selected and weighted, and based on clinical judgement or on mathematical criteria. Pooled indices, because they have a small standard deviation, are more sensitive to change than single measures. This means that smaller sample sizes are needed in order to demonstrate differences in a trial.

The disadvantage of pooled indices is that a 'single figure' can be difficult to interpret. There are also concerns over validity and practical problems such as complexity and computational difficulties.

DISEASE DAMAGE

Measures of disease damage assess the accumulated irreversible damage caused by either the disease or its treatment. Thus disease damage measures record the cumulative amount of scarring, destruction and deformity. In contrast, the effect of a disease on a patients' physical or psychological function, or quality of life, are defined as outcome criteria.

Radiological assessments

There are a variety of methods for scoring radiological damage for rheumatoid arthritis and osteoarthritis. The first method in rheumatoid arthritis was a global score based on a written description of the X-ray and described by Steinbrocker (1949). Kellgren and Lawrence (1957) published a set of standard films graded zero to four. Sharp (1971) intro-duced a separate scoring system for erosions and joint space narrowing. Sharp (1985) modified his system but it still remains very time consuming. It is the most widely used scoring system in the USA.

Larsen (1977) introduced a system which consists of comparing the patient's films with a set of standard radiographs graded zero to five. The metacarpophalangeal and proximal interphalangeal joints are scored individually, but the wrist is scored as a whole and then weighted. Larsen's system is the one most used in Europe.

There are few radiological scoring systems for inflammatory arthropathies other than rheumatoid arthritis. In spondylopathies the New York criteria for ankylosing spondylitis grade sacroiliitis, but they are usually used for disease classification rather than assessment.

In osteoarthritis the radiological assessments introduced by Kellgren and Lawrence in 1957 involve comparing the patient's films with a set of standard X-rays for each joint. The system has been demonstrated to be reproducible but is not sensitive to change. In addition it is a global score assessing osteophyte formation, joint space narrowing, subchondral sclerosis and cyst formation, and joint deformity. Attempts have been made to look at these components individually as they do not all progress at the same rate. It appears from these studies that the most appropriate radiological method varies from joint to joint.

DISEASE SEVERITY

Disease severity criteria are prognostic criteria. The patient with the most severe disease has the worst outcome. Patients with very active disease do not necessarily have the worst outcome, as they may respond to treatment. Disease severity, however, emphasises the seriousness of a feature with respect to the threat posed to overall health. Interest in the measurement of disease severity is related to the assumption that those with the most severe disease will use the most resources. However, studies from the USA across the spectrum of medical conditions have shown that, with few exceptions, the relationship between severity and cost is relatively weak.

OUTCOME MEASURES

Patients' interests and concerns are different from the doctors' view on outcomes. They need a different type of measure. In defining measurements of disease outcome, the views of those receiving treatment may be quite different from those giving treatment.

Clinicians collect information about the disease itself. Examples include the number of swollen and tender joints, the erythrocyte sedimentation rate, rheumatoid factor titres and radiological change. These provide valuable information on clinical status but are not really outcome measures.

Health assessment questionnaires help in monitoring the management of arthritis, help in deciding an appropriate treatment, and provide information on achieved outcomes.

Many of the health status measurements for outcome in rheumatoid arthritis have been tested and developed in clinical trials. Although they have a relatively broad focus it is unclear how well they would meet the requirements of other settings or the interests of groups other than clinical researchers. Health status measures should reflect short-term and longer-tem changes in rheumatoid arthritis. There is most evidence about their performance in durations under 2 years, while in practice long-term changes are of equal importance.

The most used instruments of assessment are the Health Assessment Questionnaire (HAQ) and the Arthritis Impact Measurement Scales (AIMS). These were developed specifically for rheumatoid arthritis. There are, in addition, several questionnaires developed for a range of health problems. These include the Nottingham Health Profile and the Sickness Impact Profile—so-called generic measures. Disease-specific measures do not cover all areas of interest, but do seem more sensitive to change than the generic measures.

All of the health status assessments are reliable, valid and responsive to change. The HAQ, in particular, has proved sensitive to significant clinical changes in clinical trials. In several studies, physical disability has been shown to be a strong predictor of future disability, damage and death. The HAQ and AIMS have multipurpose applications whereas the Western Ontario and McMaster Universities Osteoarthritis Index (WOMAC) is a disease-specific measure of function.

Health Assessment Questionnaire (HAQ)

Developed by Fries and colleagues in 1980 the HAQ is a measure of physical disability as assessed by eight functional categories. It has been well validated in both rheumatoid arthritis and osteoarthritis. Patient scores have a predictive value.

There is now an extensive literature showing the value of the HAQ in assessing the short-term response to treatment and as a strong predictor of future disability and premature death. It has been suggested that this self-report functional questionnaire is the most useful outcome measure to use in the outpatient clinic.

Arthritis Impact Measurement Scales (AIMS)

This multidimensional index was designed in 1980 to measure physical, social and emotional impact of different types of arthritis. It does not allow inter-disease outcome comparisons to be made. It takes longer for the patient to complete and has been less widely used in published studies.

Western Ontario and McMaster Universities Osteoarthritis Index (WOMAC)

Bellamy and colleagues, in 1988, developed this self-administered questionnaire for use in clinical trials of osteoarthritis of the hip and knee. It assesses pain, stiffness and physical disabilities. It has been shown to be responsive and reliable compared with other health status measures and has been well validated. It is a purpose-built instrument for assessing the progress of patients with osteoarthritis of hip or knee.

Laboratory assessment of disease activity

These include biochemical markers from various stages along the inflammation pathway, and markers of cartilage destruction. The erythrocyte sedimentation rate (ESR) and levels of the acute phase proteins are the most routine assessments. The ESR is still the best measure in routine practice, despite being neither sensitive nor specific for disease activity. Although C-reactive protein (CRP) is much more responsive and more specific for the acute phase response, it is just as non-specific for disease activity and more expensive. There is no convincing data to support the use of other laboratory measures to assess disease activity.

MEASUREMENTS IN CLINICAL TRIALS

Measurement procedures used in clinical trials in four common rheumatic diseases will now be examined to show differences.

Rheumatoid arthritis

Clinical outcome measures used in evaluating anti-inflammatory therapies involve: pain; morning stiffness; grip strength; patient and physician global assessment; and articular index. There have been several outcome conferences which have addressed the need for international standardisation of these measures. At the Outcome Measurement in Rheumatoid Arthritis Clinical Trials (OMERACT) conference a core set of outcome measures for phase III rheumatoid arthritis trials was proposed (Table 3.1).

Osteoarthritis

Osteoarthritis clinical trials usually examine clinical outcome measures of pain, physician global assessment and patient global assessment. A core set of outcome measures has been proposed at the OMERACT III conference (Bellamy et al., 1997). Pain, function, patient global assessment and for studies of 1 year or longer, joint imaging using validated methods and standardised techniques.

Ankylosing spondylitis

There has been no international consensus on a core set of outcome measures for phase III studies. However, the most frequently used measures have been pain, morning stiffness, chest expansion, the Schober test of forward flexion and finger to floor distance.

Fibromyalgia

There has been no international consensus on a core set of measures for phase III trials. However, the most frequent measures involve tender joint counts, patient global assessment, fatigue, quality of sleep, pain and stiffness.

MEASUREMENT IN CLINICAL PRACTICE

The success of clinic-based studies often depends on data acquired using patient self-report questionnaires, since they can be completed by the patient while sitting in the waiting room. It is important that the results are available at the time the patient is seen and the questionnaires must be short, and fit the routine of the clinic. In clinical practice, a decision must be made whether to assess all patients formally. The most obvious patients to assess are those with chronic disorders in whom long-term follow-up is indicated. The essential characteristics of a measure for use in outpatients are: simplicity, rapid completion, easy scoring, reliability, validity and sensitivity to change.

REFERENCES

Bellamy N (1993). *Musculoskeletal Clinical Metrology*. Dordrecht: Kluwer Academic Publishers.

Bellamy N, Buchanan WW, Goldsmith C et al. (1988). Validation of WOMAC: a health status instrument for measuring clinically important patient relevant outcome to antirheumatic drug therapy in patients with OA of the hip or knee. *J Rheumatol* 15: 1833–1840.

Bellamy N, Kirwen J, Boers M et al. (1997). Recommendations for a core set of outcome measures for future phase III clinical trials in knee, hip and hand osteoarthritis—consensus development at OMERACT III. *J Rheumatol* 24(4): 799–802.

Boers M, Tugwell P, Felson ET et al. (1994). World Health Organisation and International League of Associations for Rheumatology core endpoints for symptom modifying antirheumatic drugs in rheumatoid arthritis clinical trials. *J Rheumatol* 21 (Suppl. 41): 86–89.

Cuchacovich M, Couret M, Peray P, Gatica H and Sany J (1992). Precision of the Larsen and the Sharp methods of assessing radiologic change in patients with rheumatoid arthritis. *Arthritis Rheum* 35: 736–739.

Doyle DV, Dieppe PA, Scott J et al. (1981). An articular index for assessment of osteoarthritis. *Annals Rheum Dis* 40: 75–78.

Fries, JF, Spitz P, Kraumes RG and Holman HR (1980). Measurement of patient outcome in arthritis. *Arthritis Rheum* 23: 137–145.

Fuchs HA, Brooks RH, Callahan LF and Pincus T (1989). A simplified twenty-eight-joint quantitative articular index in rheumatoid arthritis. *Arthritis Rheum* 39: 531–537.

Kellgren JH and Lawrence JS (1957). Radiological assessment of OA. *Annals Rheum Dis* 16: 494–501.

Lansbury J (1988). Report of a three year study of the systemic and articular indexes in RA: therapeutic and clinical considerations. *Arthritis Rheum* 1: 505–522.

Larsen A, Dale K and Eek M (1977). Radiographic evaluation of rheumatoid arthritis and related conditions by standard reference films. *Acta Radiologica(Diagnosis)* 18: 481–491.

Melzak R (1975). The McGill Pain Questionnaire. Major properties and scoring methods. *Pain* 1: 275–299.

Ritchie DM, Boyle JA, McInnes JM et al. (1968). Clinical studies with an articular index for the assessment of joint tenderness in patients with rheumatoid arthritis. *QJM* 147: 393–406.

Sharp JT, Lidsky MD, Collins LC et al. (1971). Methods of scoring the progression of radiologic changes in rheumatoid arthritis. Correlation of radiologic, clinical and laboratory abnormalities. *Arthritis Rheum* 14: 706–720.

Steinbrocker O, Traeger CH, Batteman RC (1949). Therapeutic criteria in rheumatoid arthritis. *JAMA* 140: 659–662.

Thompson PW, Kirwan JR, Currey HLF (1988). A comparison of the ability of 28 articular indices to detect an induced flare of joint inflammation in RA. *Br J Rheum* 27: 375–380.

World Health Organisation (1980). *International Classification of Impairments, Disabilities and Handicaps*. Geneva: WHO.

Table 3.1. Core set of outcome measures for rheumatoid arthritis

Pain	Patient global assessment
Function	Physician global assessment
Number of tender joints	CRP or ESR
Number of swollen joints	Radiographs (for disease modifying studies)

Examination of specific regions

4

The shoulder

The principal function of the shoulder is to put the hand into a position where it is able to operate efficiently. Evolutionary development has been accompanied by structural changes in the shoulder girdle and its musculature. The resulting mobility has been acquired at the expense of stability and has led to complexity of soft-tissue components—ligaments, tendons and muscles. Movement is dependent on the unhampered gliding of the periarticular structures—the musculotendinous rotator cuff, the subacromial bursa and the tendon of the long head of the biceps muscles. It is the pathological changes in these structures that cause much shoulder pain.

A great deal can be learned about shoulder function from careful clinical examination and analysis of movement. Normal shoulder motion is the result of a complex of five functional areas: the glenohumeral joint, the acromioclavicular joint, the subacromial joint between the acromioclavicular arch above and the head of the humerus and tuberosities below, and the sternoclavicular and scapulothoracic region (Fig. 4.1).

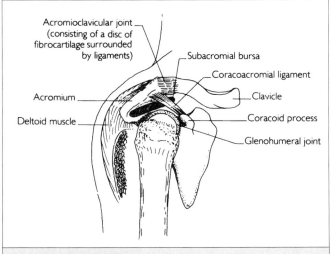

Fig. 4.1 The shoulder girdle.

Shoulder pain is one of the most common medical complaints and a detailed history and physical examination are essential to determine whether shoulder symptoms arise from local injury, or are due to occupation or systemic disease, or result from pain referred from another site. Particular attention should be given to the patient's occupation or sporting activities, and the presence of chronic illness, particularly diabetes mellitus.

Regional shoulder complaints rank fifth among the regional rheumatic diseases as a cause of incapacity or of visiting a physician. Nearly one million cases were recorded in the USA in 1976 by the National Center for Health Statistics (Kelsey, 1982). Data from UK general practices (Department of Health and Social Security, 1986) suggest that approximately one in 170 of the adult population will present to their general practitioner with a new episode of shoulder pain each year. This contrasts with one in 30 for back pain.

Arthritis of the glenohumeral joint is a relatively infrequent but important cause of shoulder pain. Although the synovial reflections of the joint are extensive, it is very difficult to identify landmarks or localise inflammation to this joint by palpation. Pain or restricted passive external rotation suggests intra-articular diseases and should not be dismissed; it may be associated with systemic disease, for example in inflammatory arthritis or infection.

Disorders of the rotator cuff tendons are common and a large proportion occur in the absence of systemic disease. In these circumstances, local causes, such as chronic repetitive low-grade trauma or excessive and unaccustomed use, either at work or at play, may be responsible. These factors may also cause partial interruption of the blood supply, resulting in incomplete attempts at healing and degeneration, which renders these tissues more vulnerable in the middle-aged and the elderly, in whom the lesions predominate. The pathological hallmarks associated with the rotator cuff syndrome include a spectrum of dystrophic changes in the tendon and accompanying calcification associated with the tendon.

ANATOMY

The shoulder joint depends very much on the surrounding soft tissues for its stability and function and the rotator cuff tendons occupy a central role. As they are the site of the majority of lesions producing shoulder pain, knowledge of their anatomy is important in understanding how such lesions may arise and why they affect shoulder function in the way they do.

The shoulder is a multi-axial spheroidal joint between the roughly spherical head of the humerus and the shallow glenoid cavity of the scapula. The shoulder is capable of a great range of movement. It is, however, a potentially very unstable type of joint compared with the hip, which has exact congruity of joint surfaces (Fig. 4.2). The glenoid labrum of fibrocartilage helps deepen the glenohumeral joint but much of the head of the humerus is still not in continuous contact with the glenoid.

Joint capsule, muscles around the shoulder

The *capsule* of the glenohumeral joint is a synovial-lined, fibrous structure that envelops the joint. It is loose and allows a 2–3 cm separation of the bones by a distractive force. The intra-articular volume enclosed by the capsule is between 20 and 50 ml. The proximal attachment is to the glenoid and root of the coracoid process, and distally to the anatomical neck of the humerus, with an extension medially 1 cm down the bone shaft. Three minor capsule thickenings, the *superior*, *middle* and *inferior glenohumeral ligaments*, help support it. Strength above is provided by the rotator cuff tendons. The *coracohumeral* and *transverse humeral ligaments*

also assist; below there is no additional support, producing a large inferior recess (Fig. 4.3). Two or three openings are present in the capsule. Anteriorly is a communication with the bursa behind the tendon of subscapularis and between the tuberosities for the longhead of biceps. Posteriorly an inconstant communication is found with a bursa below the infraspinatus.

Muscles around the shoulder joint

Superiorly lies the supraspinatus, inferiorly there is the long head of triceps, anteriorly is found the subscapularis, whilst posteriorly are the infraspinatus and teres minor. Inside passes the long head of biceps to its insertion on the upper part of the glenoid labrum. The deltoid muscle overlies these tendons. The shoulder joint capsule is fused with parts of the tendons of supraspinatus, infraspinatus, teres minor and subscapularis muscles to produce a musculotendinous cuff (the rotator cuff) (Fig. 4.4); although the tendons are fused with the capsule in the adult, they are separate in the newborn. The tendons are very small initially and become lengthened with age. The supraspinatus tendon has a mean length of 19 mm and the infraspinatus and subscapularis a length of 16 mm. The position of the rotator cuff is superiorly over the joint, separating it from the subacromial bursa (no natural communication exists between them).

The *supraspinatus* muscle is the most important rotator

Fig. 4.2 Comparison of shoulder and hip joint.

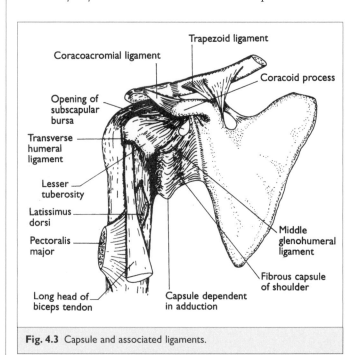

Fig. 4.3 Capsule and associated ligaments.

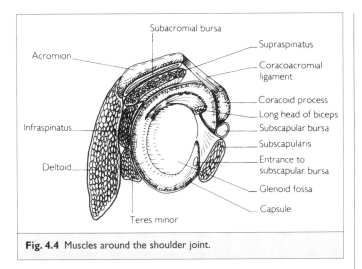

Fig. 4.4 Muscles around the shoulder joint.

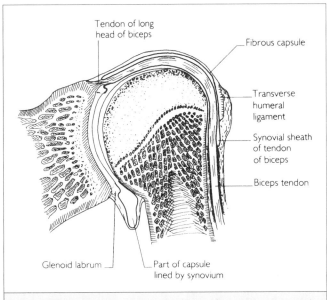

Fig. 4.5 Long head of biceps tendon and bicipital groove.

cuff muscle. Arising from the supraspinatus fossa of the scapula it inserts into the greater tuberosity of the humerus. As it passes across the superior aspect of the joint, the inferior surface of the tendon merges with the capsule, whilst the superior surface forms part of the floor of the subacromial bursa. The role of this muscle in shoulder movement is controversial: while it assists abduction by fixing the head of the humerus against the glenoid, it is not certain whether or not it is a prime mover. It is generally thought that it is mainly important in the initial 15–20° of abduction, which is otherwise mainly produced by the deltoid muscle.

The *infraspinatus* muscle has its origin on the posterior aspect of the scapula below the spine and inserts into the greater tuberosity on its posteriosuperior aspect. It is a principal lateral rotator of the humerus.

The *teres minor* has its origin along the axillary border of the scapula and inserts into the greater tuberosity on its posterioinferior aspect, at which site it is closely associated with the joint capsule and acts to strengthen it. The muscle assists the infraspinatus in its action.

The *subscapularis* muscle arises from the subscapula fossa and inserts into the lesser tuberosity of the humerus just lateral to the glenoid labrum. The bicipital groove separates it from the rest of the rotator cuff. Within the groove is the long head of the biceps, which inserts into the supraglenoid tubercle (Fig. 4.5). Often a transverse ligament is present which spans a gap between the tuberosities and forms an additional attachment for the rotator cuff. The subscapularis is important in medial rotation, especially with the humerus in the adducted position.

The rotator cuff tendons and associated capsule insert all

round the anatomical neck of the humerus, except inferiorly where only the capsule is attached. In addition to the short muscles, the other principal muscles involved in shoulder movement are the deltoid, pectoralis major, latissimus dorsi and teres major. Other muscles assist in shoulder movement, for example the triceps and the rhomboid muscles assist with shoulder-girdle movements.

Additional structures around the shoulder

The arch of the acromion covers the superior aspect of the glenohumeral joint and articulates with the clavicle at the acromioclavicular joint. The *coracoacromial ligament* is a flat band extending from the medial border of the acromion in front of the acromioclavicular joint to the lateral border of the coracoid process of the scapula (Fig. 4.6).

A number of synovial-lined *bursae* are found around the shoulder joint. There are those associated with the subscapularis and infraspinatus muscles, and in addition bursae are also present over the upper surface of the acromium and between the coracoid process on the joint capsule. Sometimes bursae are found along the long head of the triceps, the teres major and the latissimus dorsi muscles (Fig. 4.7). The largest is the subacromial bursa, which laterally is situated between the deltoid muscle and joint capsule, and medially is prolonged under the acromium and coracoacromial ligament, separating these structures from the supraspinatus tendon.

Fig. 4.6 Coracoacromial ligament.

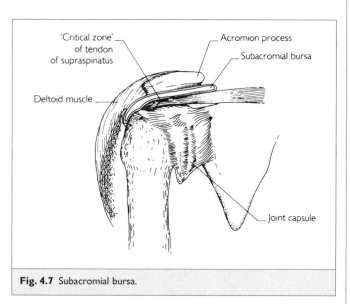

Fig. 4.7 Subacromial bursa.

Blood supply to the shoulder

The vessels supplying blood to the shoulder structures are branches of the anterior and posterior circumflex humeral arteries and the suprascapular artery.

Nerve supply to the shoulder

Two main sensory nerves supply the shoulder region. The *suprascapular nerve* supplies the superior and posterior parts of the joint and capsule and most of the rotator cuff tendon, while the *axillary nerve* supplies the anterior aspect of the joint and capsule. The axillary nerve arises from the posterior cord of the brachial plexus and exits through the quadrilateral space. This space is bordered superiorly by the teres major, inferiorly by the teres minor, medially by the long head of the triceps, and laterally by the humeral shaft and

lateral triceps heads (Fig. 4.8). After sending a sensory branch to the upper lateral cutaneous surface and a motor branch to the teres minor, the nerve courses anteriorly to innervate the deltoid.

The suprascapular nerve is a branch of the upper trunk of the brachial plexus formed by the 5th and 6th cervical nerves. It passes obliquely beneath the trapezius and crosses the scapula through the suprascapular notch (Fig. 4.9). The

Fig. 4.8 Quadrilateral space.

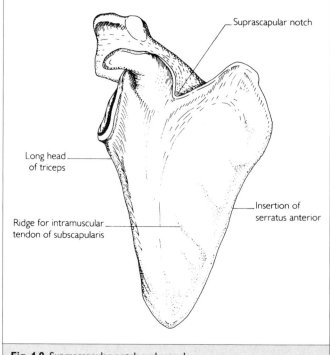

Fig. 4.9 Suprascapular notch and scapula.

suprascapular nerve has no cutaneous sensory branches but supplies motor branches to the supraspinatus and infraspinatus muscles. The acromioclavicular joint also receives branches from the suprascapular nerve but has a branch from the long thoracic nerve as well.

EVOLUTION OF THE SHOULDER

The adoption of an arboreal habitat makes the development of a highly mobile prehensile forelimb useful. The relationship of the scapula to the thorax and the orientation of the humeral head have changed with the evolution of the bipedal primates. As a strut the clavicle is an ancient possession of the vertebrates; it is a dermal bone in origin.

The groups of muscles that perform flexion, extension and adduction of the limb at the girdle show differences in development in the various primates. In quadrupedal primates the emphasis is on flexion, whereas in brachiators it is on adduction. Humans are in some features like brachiators and in others like quadrupedal primates.

DEVELOPMENTAL ABNORMALITIES

Congenital elevation of the shoulder (Sprengel's shoulder) occurs when the scapula has only partially descended from the neck of the thorax (Fig. 4.10). This may be associated with webbing or shortening of the neck.

Deformity is also seen in Erb's palsy, abduction contracture leading to a sloping deformity or secondary to kyphoscoliosis.

FUNCTIONAL ANATOMY OF THE SHOULDER

The structure of the shoulder joint allows an infinite variety of movement but is classically described as having movements of flexion, extension, abduction, adduction, circumduction and medial (internal) and lateral (external) rotation. The range of movement is greater than in any other joint. In addition, it should be noted that at rest the head of the humerus is retroverted 20–30° from the plane of the trunk; this has implications, for example flexion relative to the trunk must involve some lateral rotation.

Although the glenohumeral joint is the main articulation of the shoulder, it is not the only site of movement. Indeed, despite its greater range, movement of the glenohumeral

Fig. 4.10 Sprengel's deformity—partially undescended scapula.

joint is far less than the overall range of movement, since movement also occurs at four other sites. Scapular rotation may disguise glenohumeral stiffness (Fig. 4.11), for example. That is not to say that these occur after glenohumeral movement, but they progressively accompany it, allowing the girdle to move in a smooth rhythmic way. The soft-tissue structures of muscles, tendons and ligaments form a complex system which are as important as the bony structures. There are two other joints which also move—the acromioclavicular and sternoclavicular joints. These are true plane

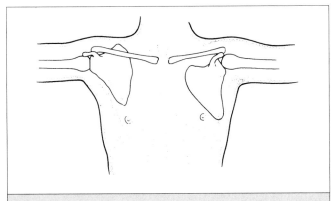

Fig. 4.11 Scapular rotation may disguise glenohumeral stiffness.

joints, but movement does also occur at two other sites which, although not structurally true joints, act like true joints. This movement is between the scapula and thoracic wall and in the subacromial region where the subacromial bursa is found. The bursa acts like a joint space separating the acromioclavicular arch and the head of the humerus. As the subacromial bursa is intimately related to the rotator cuff, the acromioclavicular joint and other nearby skeletal structures, it is often involved when these are the site of a pathological lesion.

The first 30° of abduction is achieved by contraction of the supraspinatus, the next 60° by the deltoid and the final 90° by the trapezius acting on the scapula. Adduction is principally due to the pectoralis major and latissimus dorsi. Forward flexion depends mainly on the pectoralis major and the anterior fibres of deltoid, extension on the latissimus dorsi, teres major and the posterior fibres of the deltoid. Lateral rotation is achieved by contraction of the infraspinatus and medial rotation by the pectoralis major latissimus dorsi and the anterior fibres of the deltoid.

Acute stress can result in trauma to the capsulolabral complex of the shoulder and lead to joint subluxation or dislocation (Fig. 4.12). Symptomatic instability may continue following such episodes; indeed it can develop in the susceptible individual without any history of antecedent trauma. Repeated episodes of instability place increased stress on the stabilising structures such as the rotator cuff and bicipital tendon, thereby giving rise to impingement or tendinitis. In the young athlete, development of tendinitis in the shoulder is such a frequent manifestation of an underlying instability that patients under the age of 25 with shoulder symptoms should always be assessed for the presence of glenohumeral instability.

HISTORY

General history

A painful shoulder may be seen in association with several medical conditions and it is therefore important in the evaluation of the shoulder joint to determine whether there is a relevant previous medical history. A previous cerebrovascular accident may have led to upper limb weakness, spasticity or secondary capsulitis of the shoulder joint, and pain may be referred to the shoulder from those disorders of the upper abdomen which give rise to diaphragmatic and hence phrenic nerve irritation. A Pancoast's tumour at the apex of the lung can present with shoulder-tip pain, and diabetes mellitus has a strong association with adhesive capsulitis. In addition, symptomatic involvement of other joints must be determined at the initial assessment as they may herald the onset of polyarthritis.

There is a close association between disorders of the neck and shoulder, often complicating the diagnosis, and so any history of neck pain or headaches must be recorded, as must a history of intolerance to cold or pallor of the fingers, perhaps indicating Raynaud's phenomenon or thoracic outlet obstruction. A history of previous injury or dislocation of the shoulder (Fig. 4.12) and any subsequent treatment to the shoulder is of importance, and in cases where corticosteroid injections have been administered the frequency and location of these need to be established.

Age

The age of the patient may provide clues as to the likely cause of a painful shoulder: for example, osteoarthritis and cervical spondylosis are usually conditions of the elderly. Adhesive capsulitis and degenerative rotator cuff tears tend to occur over the age of 40, and pain resulting from shoulder

Fig. 4.12 Dislocation of the shoulder.

instability is usually a condition affecting the teenager or young adult. In the case of a rotator cuff tendinitis, the pathology giving rise to the symptoms is to some extent age-related, a rough guide being underlying glenohumeral instability in the under 25-year-old, impingement or tendinitis in the 25- to 40-year-old, and degenerative rotator cuff tendinitis in the over 40-year-old group.

Arm dominance

It is important to establish handedness, as discrepancies in muscle bulk strength and range of shoulder movement may simply reflect the dominance of a particular limb.

Occupational history

Work involving heavy lifting or repetitive movements, especially above shoulder level, may give rise to tendinitis often of insidious onset. Pain is often of an aching nature and muscular in origin, often poorly localised. The patient usually notices that work aggravates or indeed precipitates the symptoms.

Pain history and sources of shoulder pain

Developmentally almost all structures of the shoulder are derived from the C5 sclerotome, at least in part. Therefore pain from any of these deep structures will be perceived in the distribution of the C5 *dermatome* (Fig. 4.13). This means that pain is localised as much to the insertion of the deltoid and outer aspect of the arm (sometimes extending to the wrist) as the shoulder itself. On the superior aspect of the shoulder is the acromioclavicular joint, which is a structure from the C4 sclerotome, so pain from here is localised to that area and not felt down the arm (Fig 4.13).

Shoulder pain may either arise from shoulder-related structures or be referred from pathology elsewhere. Local lesions producing shoulder pain may arise from the acromioclavicular joint, the glenohumeral joint itself or the periarticular structures, which the shoulder relies on for its integrity and function. It is important to establish the location of the pain and the presence of night pain or any aggravating or relieving factors. It is also important to establish whether there is associated neck pain as this may indicate the presence of pathology such as cervical spondylosis, which frequently presents with shoulder pain. Whether the onset of pain was acute or gradual should also be estab-

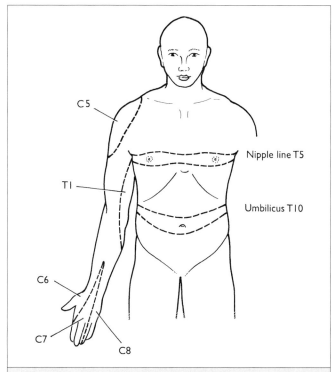

Fig. 4.13 Dermatomes around the shoulder.

lished and the relationship of pain to particular activities. Any history of injury or fall is of special relevance.

Location of pain

Pain felt at the tip of the shoulder may be referred from the subphrenic region and pain referred from the cervical spine is often maximal over the superior aspect of the shoulder (Fig. 4.14). Glenohumeral joint pathology including capsulitis and rotator cuff tears gives rise to deep-seated pain affecting the whole shoulder and often felt to come from the area of the deltoid muscle. It is aggravated by activity and relieved by rest, although it can be a problem at night. Pain from a rotator cuff tendinitis is usually felt at the outer aspect of the upper arm in the region of the deltoid insertion.

Acromioclavicular joint pathology gives rise to a well-localised pain felt at that joint and is aggravated by lying on the shoulder. Sternoclavicular joint symptoms are also well localised. If there is glenohumeral joint subluxation, pain is felt in the anterior or posterior aspect of the glenohumeral joint depending on the direction of the instability, but this is not always so. Pain that radiates up into the neck or into the forearm and hand is suggestive of a cervical or brachial plexus lesion.

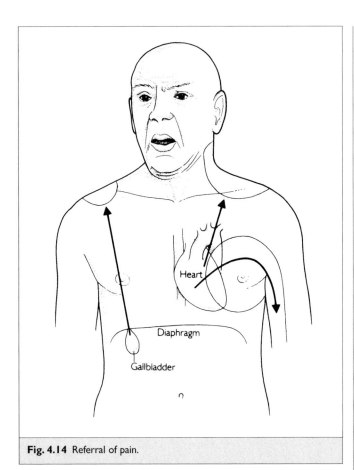

Fig. 4.14 Referral of pain.

Radiation of pain into the arm associated with numbness or paraesthesiae may indicate a compressive neuropathy, and this occurs in thoracic outlet syndrome or suprascapular or axillary nerve entrapments. The pain of a brachial neuritis is usually intense, of acute onset and has a characteristic poorly localised radiation into the arm and shoulder.

Assessing thoracic outlet compression on movement

Thoracic outlet symptoms are aggravated or brought on by activities that involve elevation of the arm. Unlike rotator cuff disorders, however, the symptoms are often aching in nature and tend to radiate into the distal arm, commonly along the ulnar border of the forearm or hand, with associated pallor, coldness or numbness of the fingers.

Axillary nerve entrapment

Entrapment as it passes through the quadrilateral space causes pain, weakness and atrophy. It is usually seen in athletes who carry out excessive overhead activity. Pain is made worse by palpation of the quadrilateral space.

Suprascapular nerve entrapment

The primary symptom is pain, which is described as a deep ache felt over the upper border and body of the scapula. It is well localised and is aggravated by any activity that brings the scapula forward, such as reaching across the chest. Palpation of the suprascapular notch is tender.

Pain located to the anterior aspect of the shoulder radiating down into the biceps muscle is suggestive of a bicipital tendinitis, especially when found in conjunction with tenderness over the long head of the biceps tendon in the bicipital groove. The tendon becomes prominent when the humerus is externally rotated.

Night pain

Shoulder pain is frequently felt at night. Capsulitis, glenohumeral joint arthritis and chronic rotator cuff tears are associated with a deep-seated constant aching pain which is made worse by changing movement and often wakes the patient. Acromioclavicular joint pathology and rotator cuff tendinitis lead to a more localised pain, which is usually felt when the patient lies on the affected shoulder. With cervical spondylosis pain tends to be less severe at night-time in contrast to pain resulting from shoulder pathology and is often relieved by wearing a soft cervical collar.

OTHER SYMPTOMS

Stiffness or loss of movement, weakness, numbness, paraesthesiae and headaches also occur with shoulder pain. Stiffness is characteristic of capsulitis and glenohumeral osteoarthritis. The stiffness is often of acute onset in adhesive capsulitis but is more gradual with degenerative arthritis. Weakness when present may be marked. It may be a true weakness or secondary to pain. It occurs rapidly in rotator cuff tears and brachial neuritis or with an entrapment neuropathy, and is mild with associated pain on attempted movement in a rotator cuff tendinitis. When weakness is due to cervical nerve root entrapment it is usually slow and progressive and associated with sensory symptoms. Swelling is not a common complaint but does occur in inflammatory conditions of the acromioclavicular or glenohumeral joints when effusion is present.

Crepitus is often described by the patient as grinding in the shoulder and may indicate subacromial inflammation or acromioclavicular joint or glenohumeral joint arthritis.

Clicks, as an isolated symptom, are not infrequent in the normal shoulder. If they are painful then they are significant and are frequently a manifestation of shoulder instability. Clicking sensation produced by certain movements may indicate a glenoid labrum tear or a subluxing biceps tendon.

Instability of the shoulder joint is common and patients may give a history of previous dislocation. Clunks are a feature of major instability. Pain is produced on certain manoeuvres, such as throwing, and there is often a feeling of a dead arm with the latter, which may last for several minutes and be followed by symptoms of rotator cuff tendinitis. Weight training, swimming and throwing sports all have a high incidence of shoulder disorders and, in many cases of glenohumeral subluxation, symptoms are often only noted during sporting activity, particularly in throwing sports.

EXAMINATION

A systematic approach is important in order to assess fully all the structures in the joints around the shoulder itself. As with other areas of the musculoskeletal system, it should include an assessment of those areas of the body where a source of referred pain is suspected, such as the upper abdomen in the case of shoulder-tip pain. The neck, axilla and chest require inclusion. Both shoulders should be examined, and any difference between the two sides noted, in terms of power, stability and range of motion, taking into the account the handedness of the patient. Neurological examination is important, particularly in cases where cervical spine disease, brachial neuritis or nerve entrapments are suspected; in addition, the peripheral pulses should be examined. Weakness is usually the predominant symptom if there is a primary neurological disorder.

Inspection

Watching the patient remove his or her shirt provides the clinician with the ideal opportunity to observe any functional limitations. Areas of erythema, discoloration, bruising and swelling should be noted. Deformity of the shoulder girdle may be present in acromioclavicular joint separation or fractures of the clavicle or humerus. Muscle wasting, which may be marked if there is cervical root or brachial plexus pathology, is less marked in rotator cuff tears or chronic tendinitis. Trapezius wasting is seen in any disorder of the shoulder which causes prolonged disuse. However, some disorders cause a disproportionate wasting, the commonest being damage to the accessory nerve in the posterior triangle of the neck. This may occur after a penetrating injury.

Like trapezius wasting, deltoid wasting is seen in all disorders that cause prolonged disuse, but may not be so obvious. Comparison with the other side usually helps confirm wasting. Lesions of the axillary nerve cause profound deltoid wasting and weakness. The commonest cause is dislocation of the shoulder, although damage to the nerve during operations on the shoulder is not rare.

Wasting of the supraspinatus or infraspinatus muscles might be noted in chronic tendinitis. Standing behind the patient, the scapulohumeral and scapulothoracic rhythm can be observed as the arms are abducted. The presence of scapula elevation should be noted as this can occur in the presence of a full range of active abduction if there is subacromial or rotator cuff inflammation. Ruptured long head of the biceps tendon can be assessed if the patient is asked to actively contract the biceps muscle (Fig. 4.15). Support the patient's elbow, flexed to 90°, with one hand. With the other, grasp the patient's wrist and ask them to pull their hand towards their shoulders, while you resist this movement. If the long tendon of biceps is ruptured, the belly of biceps appears very prominent and globular, but is in the lower, rather than middle, third of the upper arm.

In serratus anterior palsy the patient cannot stabilise the scapula. In testing serratus anterior ask the patient to push

Fig. 4.15 Examination for ruptured long head of biceps tendon by resisted active elbow flexion

against the wall with both hands and compare the two sides. The scapulae are normally held flat against the rib-cage by the action of serratus anterior. With weakness, the scapula lifts off the thorax; this is described as 'winging' of the scapula (Fig. 4.16).

Palpation

Palpation can establish the presence of any areas of tenderness, assess whether there is joint swelling or determine whether there is any joint instability. The presence of tenderness is an important feature of acromioclavicular and sternoclavicular joint inflammation and it is well-localised over the biceps tendon as it runs in the bicipital groove in cases of bicipital tendinitis. However, in the latter case, the other shoulder should also be examined as the bicipital tendon is normally sensitive to touch. There may be tenderness over the insertion of the infraspinatus, supraspinatus or sub-

(a)

(b)

Fig. 4.16 Scapular winging seen from behind (a) and from above (b).

scapularis tendon in cases of tendinitis, but in many cases of subacromial pathology no localised tenderness is found. The glenohumeral joint region and the capsular attachment should be palpated, as these areas are tender in instability. The presence of crepitus should be noted and palpation will determine whether or not this is due to inflammation of bursal structures in the subacromial space or due to degenerative changes in the glenohumeral or acromioclavicular joints. Crepitus felt at the scapulothoracic articulation may be due to scapulothoracic bursitis. Examination of the muscles of the shoulder girdle will elicit trigger points of pain, particularly present with myofascial syndromes or isolated muscle spasm.

The sternoclavicular, acromioclavicular and glenohumeral joints should all be assessed for the presence of instability when symptoms appear to be originating from these joints. In the case of the sternoclavicular joint, this can be carried out as the arm moves through full abduction. Pain and tenderness are well localised. In the normal joint the clavicle rotates through 30–40° during this manoeuvre. Excessive widening of the joint as the shoulder is retracted indicates laxity of the sternoclavicular joint capsule and its ligamentous support. Acromioclavicular joint symptoms commonly occur as a result of instability, and the joint should be examined to assess anterioposterior and inferosuperior laxity. Assessment of glenohumeral joint instability is of particular importance in the young adult presenting with shoulder pain.

When there is swelling around the shoulder it is important to establish whether the fluid lies in the subacromial bursa or in the glenohumeral joint. Communication between the two is occasionally demonstrated by milking the fluid from one compartment to the other. Swelling of the acromioclavicular and sternoclavicular joints is readily palpable and usually tender. The supraclavicular fossa should also be examined for any swelling due to lymphadenopathy or other space-occupying lesion.

Muscle testing and range of movement (Fig. 4.17)

Active and passive ranges of movement of both shoulders (Table 4.1) must be assessed and this should include assessment of abduction, adduction, forward flexion and external rotation, both with the arm by the side and at 90° of abduction (Figs 4.17–4.22). Movement is best observed from behind the patient, where the scapula can also be seen. Start

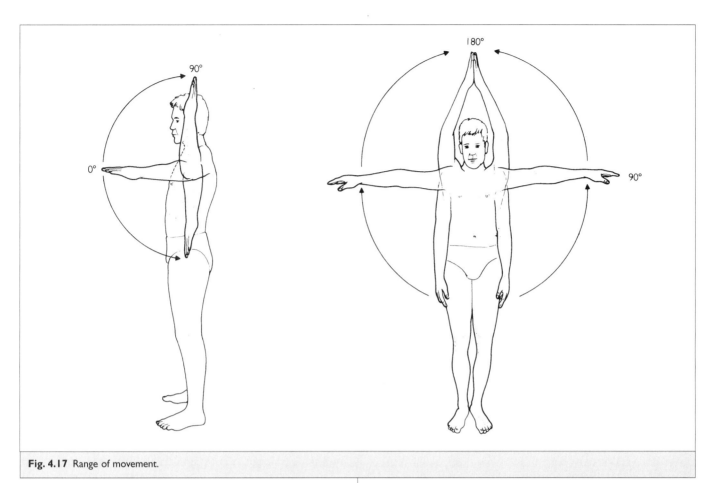

Fig. 4.17 Range of movement.

Fig. 4.18 Test for abduction (hold scapula).

Fig. 4.19 Full abduction only possible when humerus externally rotated.

with abduction, noting not only the range of movement but also the rhythm and symmetry of movement; these features are the first to be disturbed in rotator cuff disorders.

The first 90° of abduction takes place mainly at the glenohumeral joint. As the arm rises, the scapula begins to rotate on the thorax (Fig. 4.23). In the last phase of abduction movement is almost entirely scapulothoracic. True glenohumeral movement occurs only up to 90°. It can be tested (Fig 4.18) by placing a hand on the scapula, thus preventing

Table 4.1.   Range of shoulder movement

Movement	Range
Abduction	180°
Adduction	45°
External rotation	90°
Internal rotation	90°
Forward flexion	180°
Extension	50°

Fig. 4.20 Test for shoulder adduction.

Fig. 4.21 Test for shoulder flexion.

(and detecting) scapular rotation. Internal rotation is assessed with the elbow extended and the arm at the patient's side. The epicondyles of the humerus are then used as markers for the degree of motion. A combined manoeuvre of internal rotation and extension assesses functional internal rotation and can be demonstrated by asking the patient to put the affected arm behind the back, as in attempting to reach the hip pocket or undo a bra strap (Fig. 4.24). Measurement is taken by noting the level of the highest spinous process reached by the patient's thumb and comparing this with the unaffected arm.

Limitation of active and passive movement of the shoulder suggests pathology involving the *glenohumeral joint and/or capsule*. Involvement of the glenohumeral joint can occur in isolation or in conjunction with rotator cuff pathology. The latter is seen in many cases of rheumatoid arthritis.

When the glenohumeral joint is involved there is limitation of both active and passive range of movement, with pain present on movement, and increasing loss of movement as the joint pathology progresses. Abduction and elevation of the shoulder are the first movements to be lost, and the presence of an effusion should also be noted. There may be warmth and tenderness of the joint when there is inflammation, but large non-inflamed effusions are seen in an apatite-related shoulder arthropathy. Usually, other joints are involved as the shoulder is rarely involved alone in inflammatory arthritis, but the shoulder can be involved in isolation when there is a large, complete tear of the rotator cuff (Fig. 4.25). The head of the humerus subluxes in a superior direction and gives rise to an arthropathy involving the subacromial joint.

Active movement may be limited by pain or weakness, and limited active range of movement of the shoulder in the presence of a full passive range of movement of the shoulder implies a disorder of the musculotendinous structures around the shoulder, such as the rotator cuff, and pain tends to be present as a limiting factor in movement. Resisted movements of the shoulder should be tested to assess the involvement of the individual muscles. Resisted abduction should be performed with the arm at the side (Fig. 4.26) and resisted external rotation and internal rotation (Fig. 4.27) are also performed in this position with the elbow flexed to 90°. The supraspinatus muscle is best tested with the arm flexed to 30° and abducted to 90° with the arm internally rotated so that the patient's thumb points directly downwards (Fig. 4.28). Abduction from this position is then resisted by the examiner. Provided that any

Fig. 4.22 External rotation is assessed first with the arms by the patient's sides, and then with the arms abducted ('clasp your hands behind your neck').

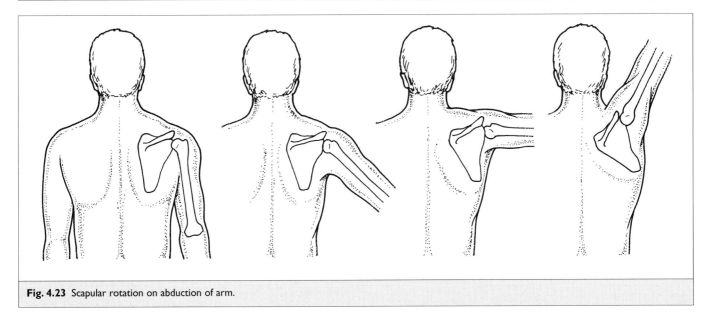

Fig. 4.23 Scapular rotation on abduction of arm.

component of adduction is eradicated, resisted internal rotation tests the subscapularis. Resisted external rotation with no element of abduction tests the teres minor and infraspinatus.

Pain on movement

The relationship of pain to movements of the arm and shoulder is helpful in diagnosis, since pain referred from the neck, thoracic lesions and intra-abdominal pathology is rarely affected by shoulder movement, whereas pain that is felt only with shoulder movement is usually due to shoulder or thoracic outlet pathology. Pain worsened by neck movement is suggestive of a cervical spine disorder.

When there is inflammation of the glenohumeral joint the pain is felt with most movements of the shoulder and pain does not disappear in full abduction and elevation as often occurs with subacromial pathology. In the latter condition,

Fig. 4.24 Test for functional internal rotation.

Fig. 4.25 Complete tear of supraspinatus tendon; the patient cannot initiate abduction. However, once the arm is lifted passively the patient can hold it abducted with the deltoid muscle.

the inflamed area is proximal to the area of impingement between the humeral head and under surface of the acromium.

There are several tests that elicit signs of bicipital tendinitis. Yergason's test involves resisted supination of the forearm with the elbow flexed at 90° and held at the patient's side (Fig. 4.29). In Speed's test the patient flexes the shoulder against resistance with the elbow extended and the forearm supinated (Fig. 4.30). Both tests are positive if pain is felt in the bicipital groove.

Painful arc of motion

Pain within a definable arc of passive or active motion is usually localised but may be diffuse. It usually indicates a mechanical disorder, such as subacromial impingement, an acromioclavicular arthritis or a rotator cuff tear. The arc of pain, in terms of both lateral and forward elevation as well as rotation, is frequently an indication of the site of the

Fig. 4.26 Resisted abduction.

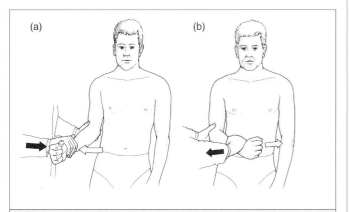

Fig. 4.27 (a) Resisted external rotation. (b) Resisted internal rotation.

Fig. 4.28 Testing supraspinatus muscle.

Fig. 4.29 Yergason's test.

Fig. 4.30 Speed's test.

pathology. If pain occurs during the entire range of gleno-humeral motion, it is likely that the source of the problem is in the glenohumeral joint itself. If the arc of pain is from 90° of abduction upwards, it is often the acromioclavicular joint that is the cause of the problem. A painful arc in the middle ranges of motion, with a painless range on either side of the painful arc, is highly suggestive of a subacromial pathology, such as a rotator cuff problem or an inferior osteophyte from the acromioclavicular joint.

Two manoeuvres stress the acromioclavicular joint and produce pain. The patient's arm is held with the elbow extended and then adducted across behind the back and pain is felt over the joint at the limit of adduction in this position (Fig. 4.31). The other manoeuvre is less specific. It involves bringing the arm across the chest under the chin with the humerus abducted at 90° from the vertical, whilst protracting the shoulder girdle (Fig. 4.32).

Symptoms of thoracic outlet compression can also be reproduced by several tests. In the costoclavicular test the patient sits with hands on thighs and thrusts the shoulder backwards in a bracing movement. Wright's manoeuvre involves abduction of the arm from 90 to 180° with the forearm externally rotated. Whilst in this position the neck is rotated to the opposite side and the patient takes a deep breath. During these manoeuvres the examiner palpates the radial pulse and a positive test is associated with a decreased or absent radial pulse. These manoeuvres,

Fig. 4.32 Testing acromioclavicular joint (second method).

although they may elicit thoracic outlet compression, may give false positive or false negative responses, and it is important to correlate any clinical findings with a reproduction of the patient's symptoms.

Assessing stability

Pain with certain movements, particularly throwing activities in the athlete, may be due to instability. Almost invariably this occurs with the arm in the outstretched (i.e. abducted and externally rotated) or overhead position. Tackling at rugby or throwing a cricket ball are common causes of acute anterior subluxation or instability, presenting as a transiently painful shoulder. The 'dead-arm syndrome' of transient numbness, tingling and weakness of the arm or hand after throwing a ball, with associated pain and later a dull ache is almost pathognomonic of shoulder subluxation. Following acute episodes there is often a history of residual pain and tendinitis lasting several days but usually responding to rest. Instability may be part of a generalised hypermobility and other joints should be examined.

Stability of the glenohumeral joint must be assessed in

Fig. 4.31 Testing acromioclavicular joint.

anterior, posterior and inferior directions. Anterior and posterior stability are best assessed with the patient standing then lying on the examination couch. With the patient standing, the examiner fixes the scapula and shoulder girdle with one hand whilst gripping the humeral head with the fingers of the other. The patient relaxes the arm by the side and the examiner can then attempt to move the humeral head forward and backward in the glenoid fossa. The degree of movement in each direction should be noted and compared with the other shoulder; any palpable clicks may indicate labral pathology.

A more accurate assessment involves the patient lying supine with the shoulder at the edge of the examination couch. The affected arm is supported by the examiner as the other hand fixes the scapula. Movement of the humeral head is then performed by direct pressure. Pain may be produced at the limits of movement. If there is a significant degree of inferior subluxation, a distinct gap can be felt between the humerus and acromium (positive *sulcus sign*). Laxity of the glenohumeral joint may be present, and further tests are required to determine whether the instability is symptomatic. The *apprehension test for anterior instability* involves the examiner attempting to extend and externally rotate the affected arm while it is held abducted 90° from the patient's side. The test is positive when there is apprehension on the part of the patient as an external rotation force is applied. With the patient lying supine on the couch and with the arm in external rotation and abduction, force can be applied to the anterior aspect of the upper humerus (Fig. 4.33). This manoeuvre often relieves any pain, and the examiner may be able to externally rotate the arm further. If the stabilising force to the anterior aspect of the humerus is removed, the patient feels pain.

Posterior instability can be assessed by stressing the posterior joint capsule, done by applying axial pressure to the forward-flexed, adducted and internally rotated arm.

Pain associated with weakness

Inability to actively abduct the arm occurs in complete tears of the rotator cuff, but usually only in large tears, and wasting of the supraspinatus and especially infraspinatus muscle is often visible and a good indicator of a rotator cuff tear. Several signs have been described to assess the degree of subacromial pathology. One impingement test involves forcing the affected arm up into full forward flexion thereby impinging the rotator cuff against the underside of the anterior acromium (Fig. 4.34). In another test, the arm is held abducted and flexed at 90° with the examiner supporting the patient's flexed elbow. With the other hand the examiner holds down the patient's shoulder girdle whilst forcibly internally rotating and elevating the affected arm (Fig. 4.35).

Cervical spine pathology

The cervical spine should always be examined when patients present with shoulder pain. This should involve assessing the range of movement, both active and passive, and assessing muscle strength, areas of muscle spasm and tenderness in the cervical and trapezius regions, and also a neurological examination. Forward flexion, extension, rotation and lateral flexion need to be assessed and any restriction in movement noted. Lateral flexion and rotation tend to be affected early in cervical spondylosis and shoulder pain resulting from cervical spine pathology may be reproduced by forced lateral flexion and rotation of the neck to the affected side.

Fig. 4.33 Stress test for glenohumeral instability. Applying pressure anteriorly relieves symptoms and allows further external rotation.

Fig. 4.34 Impingement test.

Fig. 4.36 Radiographic appearances

Fig. 4.35 Impingement test (second method).

FURTHER INVESTIGATION

Radiographs of the shoulder are frequently normal but will demonstrate any fractures or degenerative changes or soft tissue calcium around the shoulder joint. The integrity of the acromioclavicular joint may be seen and any underlying subluxation or dislocation can be reproduced with stress or weight-bearing views. The standard shoulder projection is the antero-posterior taken in recumbency (Fig. 4.36). Exam-ine the glenoid (A), the lateral border of the scapula (B), the medial border (C), its spine (D), the acromium (E) and the coracoid (F). Note the relationship of the humeral head (G) and the clavicle (H) to the glenoid and the acromium. The axial lateral view gives the most useful information, but is dependent on the patient being able to abduct the arm. It is very helpful in clarifying the relationships of the glenoid and humeral head. Arthrography of the shoulder joint is used to assess the integrity of the rotator cuff. Computerised tomography is useful in assessing pathology of the glenoid and glenoid labrum.

Arthroscopy is useful in the diagnosis of instability, sub-acromial impingement, rotator cuff tears, shoulder arthritis, synovitis and intra-articular loose bodies. Arthroscopy fre-quently adds important information to that already obtained by clinical history and examination. Direct visuali-sation of structures within the shoulder joint frequently gives information far superior to that obtained by other diagnostic procedures. This procedure led to a clearer understanding of the functional anatomy and biomechanics of the shoulder joint.

LOCAL ASPIRATION AND INJECTION

Maximum relief of pain is usually achieved with 25–50 mg of hydrocortisone acetate or equivalent corticosteroid using routine aseptic precautions.

Posterior approach

The most useful technique for non-specialised use is the posterior approach to the shoulder (Fig. 4.37). It has a good chance of success when one is not too sure of the diagnosis, as it will help in lesions of the supraspinatus, infraspinatus and subscapularis tendons, and in disorders of the glenohumeral joint.

The patient sits with his or her back to the doctor who palpates the spine of the scapula, following it laterally until it turns forward to become the acromium process, and then with the forefinger finds the coracoid process. The line between the two marks the track of the needle. If the needle is advanced 2.5 cm below the acromium process there is no resistance and the top of the needle is in the upper recess of the shoulder joint, away from the head of the humerus and the cartilage of the glenoid cavity.

Lateral approach

This is the best approach for treating a supraspinatus tendinitis (Fig. 4.38). The patient is seated with the arm loosely at his or her side; the arm is not rotated.

Palpate the most lateral point of the shoulder and advance

Fig. 4.38 Injection—lateral approach.

the needle medially below the acromium process and slightly posteriorly along the line of the supraspinous fossa. Inject when 2.5 cm of the needle is inserted. It is important that the patient does not tense the muscle, as it may then be difficult to inject.

Anterior approach to the shoulder

This approach is a little more difficult (Fig. 4.39). If the patient lies on his or her back with the forearm laid across the abdomen, the shoulder is partially internally rotated. It

Fig. 4.37 Injection—posterior approach.

Fig. 4.39 Injection—anterior approach.

is now possible to feel the coracoid process and the injection should be given just lateral to this in the direction of the joint line. Passive rotation of the arm will easily identify the head of the humerus.

The acromioclavicular joint

The joint is a plane articulation and therefore it is possible to inject it certainly from in front (Fig. 4.40). Pain arising from the joint is associated with tenderness on palpation and occasionally with swelling. The joint cavity is small and will seldom accept more than 0.5 ml of fluid. Acute lesions often settle with rest alone.

Sternoclavicular and sternomanubrial joint

With careful palpation these can be located and injected.

The glenohumeral joint

This is the true shoulder joint, and the main physical sign of glenohumeral disease is limitation of external rotation of the arm. The glenohumeral joint is best approached from the posterior or anterior aspect. The ease of injection should determine whether the needle is in the right place.

Fig. 4.40 Injection of bicipital tendon.

Injections of steroid into this joint can help the pain of the frozen shoulder and also reduce inflammation in inflammatory joint conditions.

Bicipital tendinitis

Treatment is the same as for other muscular tendinous lesions. Injection of the tendon sheath with hydrocortisone should be performed with care, as injection of the tendon may lead to rupture.

The tendon is tender and is easily palpated in the bicipital groove of the humerus. The site of maximum tenderness is marked and a needle inserted into the sheath at this mark and 0.5 ml injected. The needle is then directed superiorly along the tendon, in the sheath, for about 2 cm and more material injected. The needle is then partially withdrawn and redirected inferiorly and the remainder of the steroid injected.

Pain spots around the shoulder

Anatomical areas which are rich in pain nerve endings include the muscle–bone and ligament–bone junctions. Most pain spots around the shoulder are at these entheses. The tender areas are usually located along the scapula margin or along the spine of the scapula. They frequently respond to a weak lignocaine–corticosteroid mixture (e.g. hydrocortisone 10 mg diluted with 5 ml of 1% lignocaine). Painful tender spots around the shoulder are often referred from the neck, and in these patients the discomfort is unrelated to shoulder movements.

SUMMARY OF SHOULDER EXAMINATION

- Inspection at rest: note skin changes, swelling, wasting, deformity.
- Inspection on movement: look for painful arc; put hands behind head and back.
- Palpation: examine sternoclavicur, acromioclavicular and glerohumeral joints; look for tenderness, swelling, crepitus.
- Muscle testing and range of movement active, passive and resisted.
- Assess stability.

5

The elbow

As part of the upper limb complex, the primary role of the elbow is to permit and assist accurate spatial positioning of the hand. The elbow anchors the strong flexors and extensors of the wrist and hand, and once the shoulder has directed the hand in a gross, stable fashion, coordinated elbow movements permit fine adjustments to limb height and length. In addition, forearm rotation, at both elbow and wrist, helps place the hand in the most effective functional position.

Frequent demands on forearm muscles and poor soft-tissue protection make elbows particularly prone to enthesopathy and bursitis. The elbow is an uncommon primary target site for arthritis other than haemophilia- and syringomyelia-associated Charcot's arthropathy. Although quite commonly involved in inflammatory arthropathies (e.g. rheumatoid, psoriasis) primary osteoarthritis of the elbow, other than in the subset of pyrophosphate arthropathy, is distinctly unusual.

FUNCTIONAL ANATOMY

The elbow is a compound joint comprising three articulations: the humeroulnar and humeroradial joints (permitting flexion/extension), and the proximal radioulnar joint (which with the humeroradial and inferior radioulnar joint permits rotation; Fig. 5.1).

The humeroulnar ('trochlea') joint forms a uniaxial hinge between the trochlea of the humerus and the ulna trochlea notch. When the elbow is fully flexed (c. 145°), the longitudinal axes of the upper arm and forearm are parallel. However, due to the inclined contour of the trochlea, as the arm extends in the anatomic position (palms facing anteriorly) the long axes of the upper arm and forearm form a valgus 'carrying angle' at the elbow (Fig. 5.2). This is wider in

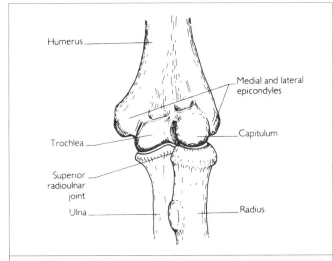

Fig. 5.1 Elbow joint anatomy.

Humerus

Medial and lateral epicondyles

Capitulum

Trochlea

Superior radioulnar joint

Ulna

Radius

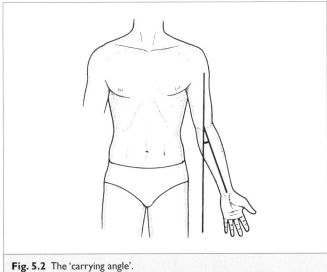

Fig. 5.2 The 'carrying angle'.

females (10–15°) than in males (5°) and may be increased—cubitus valgus—as a developmental abnormality (e.g. as part of Turner's syndrome). The opposite—cubitus varus—is a less common developmental anomaly.

The humeroradial joint is a modified uniaxial hinge (allowing rotation as well as flexion/extension) corresponding in form to a ball and socket between the capitulum of the humerus and the concave fovea of the radial head. During supination/pronation the radial head revolves on the capitulum.

The superior radioulnar joint comprises the pivot joint between the proximal rim of the radial head and the ulnar radial notch, together with the cartilage-lined annular ligament which encircles the radial head. The very strong interosseous membrane of the forearm prevents parallel displacement of the ulna and radius, and transmits longitudinal stresses from one bone to the other.

The three elbow joints share a common capsule, thus presenting an extensive synovial volume (Fig. 5.3). Both humeral epicondyles are extracapsular, but the olecranon, coronoid and radial fossae of the humerus, and the tips of the olecranon and coronoid process, are within its confines. Beneath the annular ligament the capsule extends as the sacciform recess. There are large intracapsular fat pads in each of the three fossae of the humerus which, together with muscle and soft tissues, help buttress against extremes of movement. Stability is afforded by the tight-fitting trochlear joint, the annular ligament, the cord-like radial collateral ligament and the fan-shaped ulnar collateral ligament (Fig. 5.4). The last of these has two parts which, along with flexor carpi

Fig. 5.4 Ligament arrangement.

Fig. 5.3 The synovial outline.

ulnaris, form the cubital tunnel through which passes the ulnar nerve. The capsular pattern of restriction is greater limitation of flexion than extension, with equal limitation of supination and extension.

The axis of flexion/extension runs through the humeral epicondyles: all muscles passing in front of this axis act as flexors, all those passing behind as extensors. Many of these muscles act on several joints and their action at the elbow is dependent on the attitude of neighbouring joints. The principal flexors of the elbow (Fig. 5.5) include:

- *Biceps*: joining the scapula to the radial tuberosity, thus supinating as well as flexing the elbow.
- *Brachialis*: a short muscle between the distal humerus and ulnar tuberosity, acting as a strong pure flexor.
- *Brachioradialis*: joining the lateral humerus to the radial styloid process, bringing the forearm into the neutral rotation position and then flexing the elbow.

The principal elbow extensor is the triceps, joining the scapula (via its long-head origin) and humerus (via medial and lateral heads) to the olecranon, acting to extend the elbow and swing the arm backwards (Fig. 5.6). Pronation is principally via the proximal pronator teres (the anterior interosseous nerve passes between the two heads of this muscle) and the distal pronator quadratus. Although the

Fig. 5.5 The principal elbow flexors.

Biceps   Brachialis   Brachioradialis

Fig. 5.6 The triceps.

Fig. 5.7 Extensor insertion at the lateral epicondyle.

and may rarely become compressed—*radial tunnel syndrome*—causing weakness of forearm extensors but no sensory loss). The elbow can normally undergo approximately 145° of active flexion from the fully extended position; passive flexion can often achieve another 10–15°. The elbow hyperextends 10° in many normal women (greater extension may reflect hypermobility syndrome). Individuals with well-developed muscles may lack 10° at both ends of the range.

The bones and ligaments around the elbow act to anchor the origins of the forearm muscles. The origins of the extensores carpi radialis brevis and longus (the 'fist clenchers') at the lateral epicondyle (with brachioradialis originating just above) are the usual site of pain in *lateral epicondylitis* (Fig. 5.7). Both muscles are weak elbow flexors but more importantly they extend the wrist, optimising the action of the flexors and thus permitting maximal power grip. The common tendon insertion at the medial epicondyle (for pronator teres, flexor carpi radialis, palmaris longus, flexor carpi ulnaris) is similarly the site of pain in 'medial epicondylitis' (Fig. 5.8).

Several bursae, none of which communicate with the joint, may occur around the elbow, the largest and clinically most important being the superficially placed olecranon bursa overlying the olecranon prominence.

SYMPTOMS

Pain from the three elbow compartments is usually felt maximally at the elbow close to the site of origin: severe arthropathy may cause radiation of pain down the forearm and to a lesser extent back up to the upper arm. The pain of lateral epicondylitis ('tennis elbow') is usually maximal

biceps is the strongest supinator in flexion, the supinator muscle acts in any flexion/extension position (in 30% of people the posterior interosseous nerve passes through the fibrous arcade of Frohse between the two heads of supinator

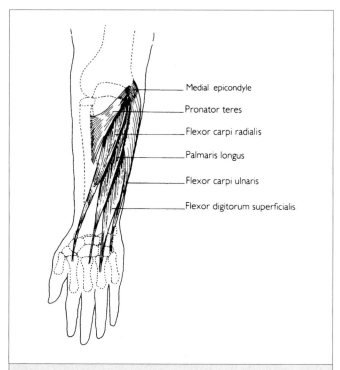

Fig. 5.8 Flexor insertion at the medial epicondyle.

- Medial epicondyle
- Pronator teres
- Flexor carpi radialis
- Palmaris longus
- Flexor carpi ulnaris
- Flexor digitorum superficialis

close to the epicondyle, radiating down the outer aspect of the forearm towards the wrist (Fig. 5.9); it is particularly marked during power grip with the wrist extended. Medial epicondylitis ('golfer's elbow') causes maximum pain around the medial epicondyle radiating down the flexor aspect of the forearm towards the wrist (Fig. 5.9). Pain from olecranon bursitis is well-localised and usually shows no

clear relationship to passive or resisted elbow movement: it may be provoked by leaning the elbow on a table, or on flexion at the elbow only when tight clothing is worn (e.g. a coat).

Four dermatomes cover sensation around the elbow (Fig. 5.10): C5/6 on the radial side and T1/2 on the ulnar side. Pain referred from above is usually ill-defined at the elbow with the site of maximum intensity elsewhere; it can be from glenohumeral or rotator cuff lesions, and from root entrapment (C5 or C6; less commonly T1, T2). Pain may be referred up towards the elbow from de Quervain's tenosynovitis, carpal tunnel syndrome or occasionally severe wrist arthropathy (particularly with a proximal synovial extension or Baker's cyst).

EXAMINATION

Inspection

Inspection from in front and behind the elbow with the patient's arm hanging by his or her side is followed by

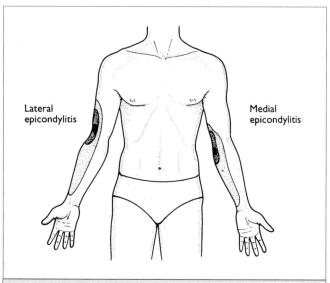

Fig. 5.9 Pain radiation in lateral and medial epicondylitis: ■ origin; ▨ site of maximum pain; ▢ area where pain is felt.

Lateral epicondylitis

Medial epicondylitis

Fig. 5.10 Dermatome distribution around elbow.

inspection during active flexion, extension and supination/pronation.

In the posterior view (Fig. 5.11) the most prominent feature is the olecranon process: para-olecranon grooves separate this from the epicondyles, the medial epicondyle being more prominent than the lateral (the three bony prominences form a straight line with the elbow extended). Anteriorly the triangular cubital fossa (Fig. 5.12) forms a hollow bounded superiorly by the biceps and its tendon, medially by the pronator teres and the common flexors, laterally by the brachioradialis, and the floor comprising the brachialis muscle and tendon (plus joint capsule and supinator). The fossa contains the brachial artery and veins, the median and musculocutaneous nerves, and superficially the median cubital vein (joining the medially placed basilic to the cephalic vein).

Inspect the skin for erythema (confined to bursitis or over the whole joint), scars and other changes, including psoriasis (the extensor aspect is a common site). The extensor forearm surface and olecranon are also common target sites for nodules and pressure sores (Fig. 5.13).

Synovial swelling may be apparent over the radial head anteriorly, and posteriorly over the paraolecranon grooves (medial < lateral). With marked synovitis the whole elbow region may appear swollen. Olecranon bursitis produces localised smooth swelling around the olecranon prominence (Fig. 5.13); nodules within it may produce a lumpy contour.

As the patient actively flexes and extends the elbow, the main deformities to look for are fixed flexion (inability to fully extend the elbow), cubitus valgus or varus (assessed with the elbow extended), and posterior subluxation of the olecranon on the humerus. The resting attitude may suggest the degree of discomfort or presence of joint disease. A capsular pattern of restriction usually affects flexion more than extension, with supination/pronation affected last: in the presence of synovitis/effusion the patient is therefore most comfortable with the elbow positioned in flexion (*c.* 45–70°).

Ask the patient to supinate and pronate the hands with the elbows tucked into his or her side at 90° flexion (Fig. 5.14). If the proximal or distal radioulnar joints, or the humeroradial joint, are compromised these movements may be painful and/or reduced (usually equally): the patient

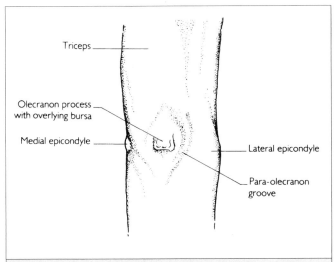

Fig. 5.11 Posterior view of the elbow: surface anatomy.

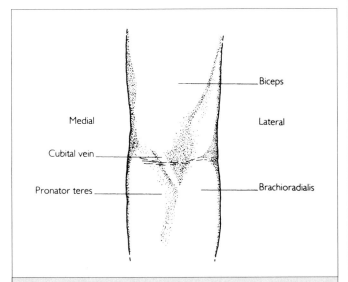

Fig. 5.12 Anterior view of the elbow: surface anatomy.

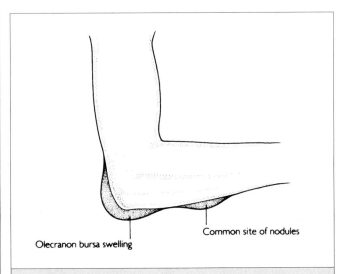

Fig. 5.13 Sites of nodules and olecranon bursa swelling.

Fig. 5.14 Forearm supination (a) and pronation (b).

often undertakes a trick manoeuvre, adducting the elbow across the abdomen to rotate the ulnar and thus increase supination.

Palpation

The elbow is conveniently palpated with the examiner standing behind the patient with the patient's shoulder extended so that the elbow points backwards in mild flexion (Fig. 5.15). Pass the back of the hand over the extensor surface of the distal upper arm, elbow and forearm to feel for increased temperature over the paraolecranon grooves and olecranon bursa. The landmarks of the medial and lateral epicondyles are easily felt. On the medial side, feel for the ulnar nerve below the epicondyle for thickening and disproportionate tenderness (this is the commonest site for ulnar nerve entrapment). The medial supracondylar lymph nodes may be palpable if enlarged. Palpate for nodules (even if not immediately apparent) along the extensor forearm border. Palpate for swelling of the olecranon bursa with the arm in extension: if the arm goes into flexion the bursa will become more tense and prominent. A balloon sign will

confirm a moderate to large fluid collection. Synovitis will produce soft-tissue swelling in the two paraolecranon grooves, particularly on the medial side: firm palpation at these sites may produce capsular tenderness.

Place a thumb and two fingers of one hand over the olecranon, medial epicondyle and lateral epicondyle. In extension the three fingers will form a straight line, whereas in flexion the fingers will form the points of an equilateral triangle (Fig. 5.16). Loss of such symmetry on flexion implies loss of height at the elbow due to cartilage and bone attrition ('triangle' sign). Place a finger in each paraolecranon groove to feel for crepitus from the humeroulnar and humeroradial joint while the patient flexes or extends.

Coming to the front of the patient, palpate over the radial head region for soft-tissue swelling due to synovitis. Occasionally palpable anterior synovial extensions may almost fill the cubital fossa (predisposing to partial radial nerve palsy due to pressure on the posterior interosseous nerve). Pressure over the radial head may produce capsular/joint-line tenderness and, if there is associated joint damage and annular ligament laxity, there may be excessive movement of

Fig. 5.15 Palpation from behind with elbow mildly flexed.

Fig. 5.16 The 'triangle' sign.

Additional tests

Tennis elbow (lateral epicondylitis): palpate over the common extensor origin at the lateral epicondyle. This may produce marked tenderness: in some cases tenderness is more distal occurring over the radial head region. Confirmation is by resisted active wrist extension which reproduces the pain of which the patient complains (Fig. 5.18).

Golfer's elbow (medial epicondylitis) frequently gives tenderness over the medial epicondyle at the insertion site of the wrist flexor/pronator group (pronator teres, flexor carpi radialis, palmaris longus, flexor carpi ulnaris). Resisted active wrist flexion with the hand supinated will reproduce the pain (Fig. 5.19).

the radial head with crepitus. Keeping the thumb over the radial head region, passively supinate and pronate with the other hand (thumb placed over ulnar styloid region) to detect crepitus (both joints) and assess the range of passive movement, and enquire concerning pain (Fig. 5.17). Pass the back of the hand down the flexor aspect of the distal upper arm, elbow and forearm, again feeling for increased temperature, particularly over the radial head region. The range of passive flexion and extension is assessed (looking particularly for restriction ± stress pain) and compared with active movements; similar restriction suggests synovitis, a greater passive range favours a neuromuscular rather than joint cause.

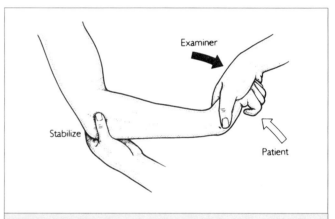

Fig. 5.18 Resisted active wrist extension (reproducing pain of lateral epicondylitis).

Fig. 5.17 Palpation of proximal and distal radioulnar joints during supination/pronation.

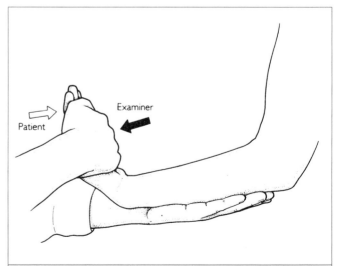

Fig. 5.19 Resisted active wrist flexion (reproducing pain of medial epicondylitis).

Collateral ligament stability may be tested as follows. Flex the patient's elbow to *c.* 20–30° and, holding the elbow in one hand, apply a progressive varus force (to test the lateral ligament) and then a valgus force (to test the medial ligament) on the distal forearm (Fig. 5.20), noting any pain or increased lateral movement.

Muscle power, if required, can be assessed by resisted active movements with the patient's arm adducted to the side and the elbow positioned at 90°. Firmly holding the elbow with one hand and the distal forearm with the other (power grip) ask the patient to:

1. *push out in extension*—principally triceps (radial nerve, C7), and then

2. *pull upwards to the shoulder in flexion*—principally biceps and brachialis (both musculocutaneous nerve; C5/6); still holding the elbow, grasp the distal forearm along its longitudinal axis and ask the patient to:

3. *supinate against resistance*—principally biceps (musculocutaneous nerve; C5/6) and supinator (radial nerve; C6); and then

4. *pronate against resistance*—principally pronator teres (median nerve; C6), and pronator quadratus (anterior interosseous branch; C8/T1).

Nerve entrapment may affect the ulnar (most common by far), median or radial nerves. Helpful tests include:

● *Tinel's sign*: light, rapid percussion over the ulnar nerve as it travels through the medial paraolecranon groove produces tingling in an ulnar distribution in the forearm/hand distal to the point of compression (Fig. 5.21). The most distal point at which the abnormal sensation is felt can be used to indicate the limit of nerve regeneration (serial testing can therefore crudely reflect rate of regeneration).

● *Elbow flexion test*: the patient holds the elbow in full flexion for 5 minutes. Tingling in an ulnar distribution again suggests a cubital tunnel syndrome.

● *Pinch grip test*: the patient attempts to oppose the tips of the index finger and thumb. If the normal tip-to-tip pinch is replaced by a pulp-to-pulp pinch (Fig. 5.22), reflecting impairment of index finger and thumb flexors, entrap-

Fig. 5.20 Testing collateral ligament stability.

Ulnar nerve

Fig. 5.21 Tinel's sign.

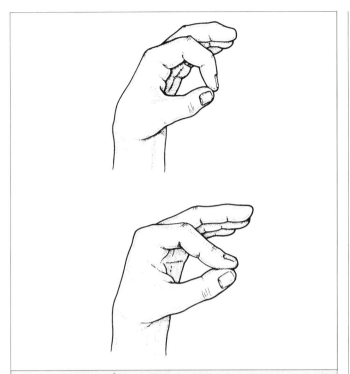

Fig. 5.22 The pinch grip test: upper, normal pinch; lower, abnormal pinch.

ment of the anterior interosseus nerve (a branch of the median nerve) as it passes between the two heads of pronator teres is suggested (*anterior interosseous nerve syndrome*). If the median nerve is compressed just prior to the anterior interosseous division, the flexor carpi radialis, palmaris longus and flexor digitorum muscles are also weak (*pronator teres syndrome*). In both cases, there is sensory impairment in a median nerve distribution. Rarely (1% of people), the median nerve is compressed as it passes (± the brachial artery) beneath the ligament of Struthers, an anomalous band running from a spur on the humerus to the medial epicondyle: in this case (*humerus supracondylar process syndrome*) the pronator teres is also involved (± vascular, as well as neurological, symptoms).

LOCAL ASPIRATION AND INJECTION

Elbow joint

The two easiest approaches to the joint are anterolaterally and posteriorly. With either approach, fluid aspiration and ease of injection both confirm correct positioning.

Anterolateral approach, towards the humeroradial joint line

Fluid usually accumulates earliest and most prominently anteriorly around the radial head (large synovial extensions, particularly in rheumatoid arthritis, may indeed expand anteriorly to fill much of the cubital fossa). With the patient's elbow resting on a firm comfortable surface, and held flexed at 90°, palpate the head of the radius while passively supinating and pronating the patient's forearm. The joint line should be readily identified, and associated soft-tissue/fluid swelling is commonly palpable at this site. Pass the needle tangentially in towards the joint line from a superolateral angle (Fig. 5.23), aiming to place the tip just within the capsule rather than deep between the two bones.

Posterior approach, towards the olecranon fossa

Fluid also expands posteriorly to cause swelling that may be apparent in the paraolecranon grooves (medial > lateral). Again, with the patient's elbow flexed to 90° and comfortably supported, identify the olecranon process (receiving the indistinctly felt triceps tendon), the paraolecranon grooves and the olecranon fossa. Insert the needle above the superior aspect of the olecranon, slightly to the lateral side, just into the olecranon fossa (Fig. 5.24).

Lateral epicondylitis ('tennis elbow')

Injection is into the site of maximal tenderness. In the majority of cases this is the anterior part of the epicondyle at the extensor carpi radialis brevis origin; less commonly it is the supracondylar crest (exensor carpi radialis longus origin), or more distally where extensor carpi radialis brevis overlies the radial head (Fig. 5.25). The patient is positioned with the

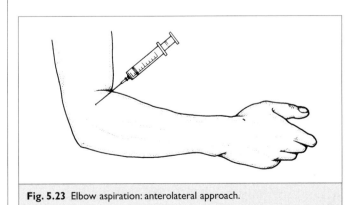

Fig. 5.23 Elbow aspiration: anterolateral approach.

Fig. 5.24 Elbow aspiration: posterior approach.

Fig. 5.25 Injection sites for lateral epicondylitis.

Medial epicondylitis ('golfer's elbow')

The situation is very similar to lateral epicondylitis. Position the patient in the same way, and identify the site of maximal tenderness (usually just distal to the medial epicondyle). After warning the patient of probable pain exacerbation, the injection is again made under pressure using a fan technique; a lesser volume of non-fluorinated steroid and lignocaine (1–3 ml) will usually suffice. The ulnar nerve runs behind and below the medial epicondyle and careful siting of the injection is therefore required.

Olecranon bursitis

The bursa is superficial and no important structures traverse its surface. Aspiration is therefore straightforward, the needle being aimed towards the site of maximal distension. Non-fluorinated steroid should be used for injection.

SUMMARY OF ELBOW EXAMINATION

- Inspection at rest: note skin changes, swelling (synovitis, bursitis, nodules), attitude, deformity (valgus, varus, fixed flexion, posterior subluxation).
- Inspection during movement: look for reduced and/or painful flexion/extension, supination/pronation.
- Palpation
  (1) from behind:
  warmth
  paraolecranon grooves (swelling, tenderness, crepitus, deformity, palpable ulnar nerve, enlarged nodes)
  olecranon region (bursa, nodules)
  (2) from in front
  warmth, swelling
  radial head (proximal radioulnar joint) tenderness, crepitus, laxity
  passive movements—supination/pronation, flexion/extension periepicondylar tenderness
- Additional tests
  resisted active wrist extension (lateral epicondylitis)
  resisted active wrist flexion (medial epicondylitis)
  instability (varus/valgus force)
  muscle power (resisted active movements)
  peripheral nerve entrapment tests (Tinel's, elbow flexion, pinch grip).

forearm supported and the elbow in mid flexion. Having identified the maximally tender site, the needle is aimed vertically downwards until it touches bone. Slightly withdraw the needle, then infiltrate both deeply (as near as possible to bone) and more superficially using a fan technique of half-withdrawals and reinsertions. The injection must be made under pressure (the one exception to the rule). Conventionally 1–2 ml is injected, although some prefer larger volumes (2–5 ml) to ensure adequate delivery. Fluorinated steroid should be avoided at this superficial site, the usual choice of injection being hydrocortisone (or methylprednisolone) in 1% lignocaine. The injection is commonly painful, and the patient should be warned that pain may be exacerbated for 24–48 hours.

6

The hand

The examination of the hand considers two issues. Are there signs of systemic disease? Are there abnormalities of the hand mechanism itself? There is no single way to examine the hand. The emphasis of the approach will depend on the problem being considered. This will be established in the history. An understanding of how the hand works helps develop the examining technique.

FUNCTIONAL ANATOMY

It seems rather simplistic but the hand is a mechanism on the arm that grips and feels. We use it to explore our environment and communicate by touch and sign. We use it to manipulate and use tools. Although several types of grip have been described the primary grips are a power grip, claw or hook and precision grip.

The hand is articulated on the arm. It is positioned in space and works on the arm. Function is therefore dependent on the integral action of the arm including the elbow and shoulder. The hand is powered by muscles in the forearm. It is a set of joints organised in rays corresponding to the digits, four fingers and thumb, which in turn articulate, through the complex set of bones making up the wrist, on the arm.

The wrist joint is a complex of small carpal bones that articulate with the distal radius and ulna and the metacarpals. Their articulation allows movement and stability. For most use the wrists is held stable in dorsiflexion. Movement in the thumb and fingers works the hand. The power to move the components of the hand is in the forearm—a set of muscles that allow extension, flexion, abduction and adduction of the wrist and digits. The interphalangeal joints are constrained so movement is primarily flexion and extension. The thumb base articulating at the scaphotrapezoid and carpometacarpal joint can rotate. The metacarpophalangeal joints have limited rotation.

Anatomy allows the hand to vary between a power and precision instrument. Maximal power grip is achieved by dorsiflexion and abduction of wrist and flexion with adduction or ulnar drift of the fingers. The relative shortening of the metacarpals across the hand to the ulnar side and the limited rotation of the metacarpophalangeal joint allows the hand to form a power grip. The phalanges close against the thenar eminence. Precision grip requires a stable dorsiflexed wrist and is primarily achieved with slight rotation in flexion of the index to allow the pulp of the index to meet the pulp of the opposing thumb.

The muscles are controlled through branches of three nerves, the radial, ulnar and median. The sensory supply to the hand is very sensitive and reflects the role of the hand as a device to sense the environment. It is supplied via three sensory roots, C6, 7 and 8.

The arterial supply is through two main arteries, the ulnar and radial, which form deep and superficial arcades that give digital arteries to the fingers and thumb.

PAIN PATTERNS

Pain is a major symptom of problems in the hand. Analysis of the pattern of pain is important in formulating questions that then are assessed in the examination. In the history establish the components of the pattern: distribution temporally and spatially, when the pain came on, how it varies, where it is. Establish worsening and alleviating features as well as any associated problems. Pain may either be focal or referred.

Referred pain is usually from a problem in the arm or neck. Often it is associated with problems in the nerve supply to the hand. Lesions of the nerve roots, the brachial plexus and peripheral nerve may all manifest as hand pain. Involvement of sensory nerve roots gives referred pain in a dermatome distribution. This will contrast with the pattern of peripheral nerve involvement which corresponds to the sensory distribution of the nerve. However, there is considerable anatomical overlap and variation that may make the clinical presentation less clear than the anatomy would suggest.

Pain from problems in the hand will primarily be from problems of infection, inflammation, trauma, degeneration or mechanical derangement or ischaemia. Features in the history will direct the examiner to possible causes. The nature of the pain is important. Intense throbbing pain interfering with sleep suggests acute inflammation of infection. Pain worse with hand use eased by rest may be associated with joint disease but raises the possibility of ischaemia. Inflammation is often worse in the morning, in contrast to pain from degenerative change, which worsens with use and the progress of the day. Pain from joint derangement such as from meniscal tears or tendon lesions may be focal and associated with particular actions using the joint.

Focal pain associated with tenderness highlights the probability of a local problem. For example, joint pain associated with morning stiffness and tenderness over the joint line or in soft-tissue swelling will focus the diagnosis on an arthritis. Diffuse pain associated with paraesthesia may be caused by a peripheral neuropathy.

There are also unusual causes of pain. Sympathetic pain, sometimes referred to as reflex algodystrophy or Sudeck's atrophy, is associated with changes in the sympathetic nervous system. It may be spontaneous or triggered by trauma. It often seems disproportionate to the severity of the injury and has been described following minor trauma. It characteristically has a burning character termed causalgia. In addition, there may be changes in blood vessel control producing Raynaud's or acrocyanosis. There may be changes in the sensory system producing hypersensitivity or algodynia. The process seems to go through a phase of activity with marked swelling and warmth and go on to be more associated with a cold hand that may develop secondary atrophic features.

A second unusual pain is associated with hypertrophic osteodystrophy. This is a painful periostitis that can be noted by tenderness around the joint, on the bone, in contrast to pain along the joint line characteristic of an arthritis.

A third difficult group of problems with hand pain are related to use. The concept of a repetitive strain injury hypothesises that repeated use sets up a pattern of pain that is persistent even after the triggering use has stopped. The problem is controversial. Repetitive use can give tenosynovitis and trauma can produce secondary degeneration, so use is linked to hand pain problems. The odd pain syndromes such as algodystrophy and phantom pain demonstrate that the mechanisms of pain remain unclear and raise the possibility that other causes of hand pain may occur.

Finally, many patients have atypical pain. The features are inconsistent with known anatomy or identifiable abnormality. There is much discussion as to the basis of this type of pain and a psychological aetiology is often supposed. In conversion phenomena a feature is the lack of insight into the underlying psychological problem by the patient. The psychological problem is suppressed and manifests as a pain problem. Inquiry may identify psychological factors. This brings out the more challenging aspects of clinical medicine. Analysis may require repeated patient assessment. The key is to keep an open mind and appreciate that medicine remains an uncertain science.

EXAMINATION

The examination of the hand is based on questions that have been suggested by the history. Is the problem about systemic disease or about functional aspects of the hand? The former may mean key signs are needed, rather than a full assessment. For example, in respiratory disease clubbing needs to be looked for but the examination otherwise will be a quick screen. In an arthritis not only is information about the type of arthritis and its complications sought but an evaluation of the functional disability is also needed.

Examination is by observation, then looking at movement and touching. It begins as the patient comes into the room and cues are given as the subject is watched using their hands, gesticulating and undressing. The formal examination is primarily by looking. Most people have a strong instinct to start touching and as soon as they do this they will be drawn away from the most important source of information and become confused by the limitations of touch.

It is best to examine the hands both together, at rest, with the patient comfortable, either sitting with the hands supported by a pillow or lying with them resting on the abdomen. Initially, look at the dorsal aspect, then ask the patient to pronate the hands and look at the volar aspect. Deliberately look proximally to distally. Look at the structure and consider whether features of systemic disease are present. Consider the skin, the overall structure and observe if there is any deformity. The pattern of deformity is particularly important. Look also for movement. Some tremor is normal, but accentuated tremor may occur in benign essential tremor, anxiety and hyperthyroidism. There may be a flap in respiratory failure and liver disease. During the examination consider the component structure: the skin, bones and joints, muscles, tendons, nerve. The skill is to be thinking of all these at once. Initially think component through each in turn.

The skin

The skin is thicker on the palmar than on the dorsal surface. It is tethered to the deeper structures at the skin creases and in the fingers to the lateral and medial ligaments of Cleland and Grayson. Loss of sweating may indicate nerve damage. The skin may be thin and bruised. There may be solar keratoses or other rashes. Eczema characteristically affects the flexures. The rash of scabies occurs between the fingers. The skin becomes atrophic in Sudeck's. In scleroderma it thickens and tightens. There may be the changes of vasculitis such as splinter haemorrhages. There may be livedo reticularis. The nails may be dystrophic, with pitting or onycholysis. On the volar aspect tightening of the palmar fascia with bands into the little and ring finger that can cause flexion contracture is due to Dupuytren's contracture (Fig. 6.1). In connective tissue diseases there may be changes in the capillary pattern at the nail bed. With magnification such as

× 20 on an ophthalmoscope they can be seen as an arcade laid flat. Increased tortuosity of vessels and areas of loss suggest a connective tissue disease is developing. Other features of this may be pulp atrophy and nodules from calcification. Nodules may also develop in rheumatoid arthritis.

Bones and joints

Consider the overall appearance of the hand. Is there a deformity? Long thin fingers may suggest Marfan's syndrome. Short fat fingers occur in achondroplasia. Shortened little and ring fingers occur in Down's syndrome and pseudohyperparathyroidism. Large hands may result from acromegaly or hypothyroidism.

The organisation of the bones in the wrist is complex but a number of landmarks can be defined (Fig. 6.2). On the radial side of the wrist the radial styloid can be felt and distally the palpating finger will cross the radiocarpal joint, naviculo-trapezial joint and finally the trapezo-metacarpal joint at the base of the thumb. The ridge in the middle of the dorsum of the radius, Lister's tubercle, runs down to the base of the middle finger along which a palpating finger crosses the radio-lunate, lunate-capatate and capatate

Flexion contracture of little finger PIP is a common idiopathic finding
Thickened palmar aponecrosis
Progressive flexion contractures of ring finger

Fig. 6.1 Dupuytren's contracture.

Fig. 6.2 The bones of the carpus (volar view). First row: S, scaphoid; L, lunate; P, pisiform; Tq, triquetrum. Second row: Tm, trapezium; Td, trapezoid; C, captitate; H, hamate. R, radius; U, ulna.

metacarpal joint. On the ulnar side of the joint a line from the ulnar styloid crosses the triquetrium and hamate to the base of the fifth metacarpal. Inferiorly the prominences of the pisiform and the hook of the hamate can be located. The latter bounds the canal of Guyon.

Passive movement of the hand allows the bones and joints to be more easily felt and local tenderness defined. Try to identify if this is periarticular or around the joint line. In hypertrophic osteodystrophy it tends to be periarticular, often around the distal radius, and is less prominent on the joint line. Early synovitis of the metacarpophalangeal joints may be first shown by squeezing across the metacarpals to elicit tenderness. Loss of movement is difficult to assess and document precisely. The wrist can flex laterally, medially and volar flex and dorsiflex or extend. It can combine this so the joint can rotate. The metacarpals and interphalangeal joints primarily flex from neutral. The metacarpal joints can laterally flex and rotate slightly. Ranges of movement in adults are shown in Table 6.1. Ranges of movement are greater in young people and in some ethnic groups. When there is hyperlaxity the metacarpal joint can dorsiflex beyond 90° and the thumb will passively extend back to touch the radius.

Patterns of deformity are particularly important in defining types of arthritis. Is the involvement symmetrical or asymmetrical? Is it predominantly distal or proximal? These features are summarised in figures (Figs 6.3–6.5). Rheumatoid arthritis predominantly involves the metacarpophalangeal joints and wrists. Psoriasis and osteoarthritis tend to involve the distal interphalangeal joints. Gout may cause an asymmetrical oligoarthritis and tophi may be apparent. Note if the swelling is soft tissue or bony and if it is tender. The wrist may sublux producing bowstringing of the extensor tendons. This may be misinterpreted as small muscle wasting. The integrity of the first dorsal interosseous muscle is important to clarify this. If it is wasted a muscle disease of

Table 6.1. Normal range of joint movement (degrees) in the hand

	Flexion	Extension	Abduction	Adduction
Fingers				
MCPs	90	30–45	20	20*
PIPs	100	0	0	0
DIPs	90	10	0	0
Thumb				
MCP	50	0	70	0
IPJ	90	20	0	0
Wrist	80	70		

(Ulnar deviation 30°, radial 20°)

*In extension but not in flexion.

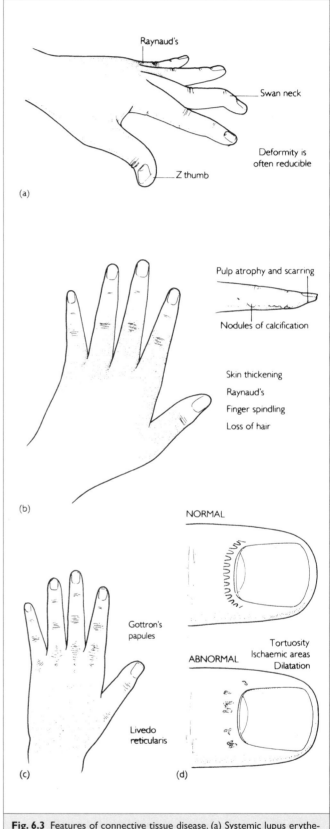

Fig. 6.3 Features of connective tissue disease. (a) Systemic lupus erythematosus. (b) Systemic sclerosis. (c) Dermatomyotosis. (d) Nail-fold changes in capillaries (seen on magnification).

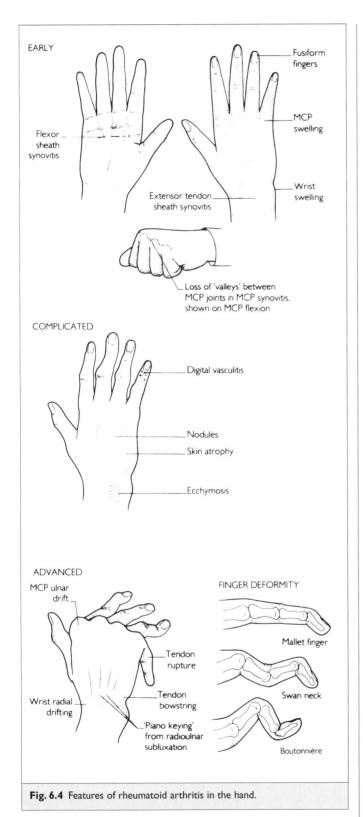

Fig. 6.4 Features of rheumatoid arthritis in the hand.

Fig. 6.5 Patterns of joint involvement in different types of arthritis.

interphalangeal joints. Initially these may be tender, soft and only later become less painful but become hard. They may be associated with hyaluronic acid cysts that are soft-tissue swellings near the joint. Often the carpometacarpal joint of the thumb is involved in osteoarthritis; then the thumb tends to rotate toward the palm of the hand and there is squaring of the base of the thumb. However, in other associated diseases and in secondary osteoarthritis involvement

T1 origin including an ulnar nerve lesion is possible.

Osteoarthritis may be primary or secondary. Bone osteophytic changes are characteristic. Involvement is predominantly distal. Nodes form in association with the distal can be more proximal. In erosive osteoarthritis greater asymmetrical interphalangeal joint involvement is seen. In pyrophosphate disease and in haemochromatosis more wrist and metacarpophalangeal joint involvement occurs. Muscle wasting may be secondary to joint disease.

Tendons and muscles

Assessment of the tendons of the hand requires an understanding of the anatomy. Consider the flexors. There are three sets: flexors of the wrist, of the digits and the flexors in the small muscles of the hand. There are two sets of long flexor tendons of the digits, sublimis and profundus. Profundus goes through a divide in sublimis to the distal phalanx. There are two sets of extensors—of the wrist and the digits. The extensor tendon of the digits forms a dorsal expansion over the top of the fingers with insertions from lumbricles and inserts itself in a central slips to the middle phalanx and lateral slips to the distal phalanx. Rupture of the slips to the distal phalanx gives a mallet finger deformity because the flexor is unopposed. Acute rupture will show absent active but present passive movement. After time the fibrosis that occurs may restrict passive movement.

In inflammatory arthrtitis, particularly rheumatoid, several named deformities may be found. In swan neck deformity the metacarpophalangeal joint and distal interphalangeal joint are flexed and the proximal interphalangeal joint is hyperextended. In the contrasting boutonnière deformity, the proximal interphalangeal joint is flexed and the distal interphalangeal joint is hyperextended. A 'Z' deformity of the thumb may result from hyperextenion of the interphalangeal joint and flexion of the proximal interphalangeal joint.

Palpation of the tendon in tension allows the integrity of the tendon to be established. Swelling of the tendon may result from tenosynovitis. This may be tender with inflammation of the synovial sheath. Tenosynovitis of the long muscles of the thumb is common and is often described as de Quervain's. Tenderness is seen over the radial tubercle in extensor pollicis longus and abductor pollicis longus. They can be seen more clearly when the thumb is extended. Finkelstein's test makes this more apparent. The subject makes a fist with the thumb tucked under the fingers. The wrist is then passively flexed and ulna deviated to stretch the tendon against the radius. If it is inflamed this will cause pain.

On the volar aspect of the wrist other tendons can be identified by asking the patient to make a fist and palpating

extensor carpi radialis longus and brevis as they pass under extensor pollicis longus. The extensor pollicis longus then passes round the ulnar styloid and turns 45° to the thumb. As the fingers are extended the tendons of extensor indicis, digitorum communis and digiti minimi can be felt. Extensor carpi ulnaris runs in a groove below the ulnar styloid and can be felt as the wrist deviates to the ulnar side.

On the palmar aspect of the hand the palmaris can be made prominent as the wrist flexes against resistance. Flexion with radial deviation makes the tendon of flexor carpi radialis prominent. The flexor sublimis and profundus are evaluated by holding the fingers in extension to allow only the action of the distal interphalangeal joints, if the produndus is intact. If three fingers are held in extension the fourth will be able to flex at the proximal interphalangeal joints if the sublimis tendon to that finger is intact.

The lumbricles arise from the flexor digitorum profundus tendon and pass across the metacarpal joints to insert into the lateral slips of the extensor expansion. Flexing the metacarpophalangeal joint and extending the interphalangeal joints demonstrates that the lumbricles are intact.

Assessing muscle power confirms that tendons are functioning and establishes if there is nerve or muscle weakness. Finger extensors are assessed by asking the subject to resist metacarpophalangeal joint extension by the examiner. Small muscle power involves assessing power of the Interco and muscles of thenar, and hypothenar eminence. It is important in establishing if there is a T1 root or ulnar nerve lesion. Abduction is assessed by the subject resisting the observer's attempt to adduct the fingers. Finger adduction is assessed by the subject trying to hold a piece of card between the fingers as the examiner pulls it away (Figs 6.6, 6.7).

Thumb movements may cause confusion because the

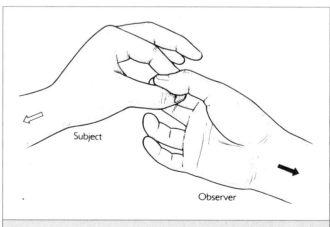

Fig. 6.6 Testing the 'O ring' in opposition of thumb and index.

Fig. 6.7 Testing finger adduction power.

thumb is rotated in relation to the hand and so has a different plane of movement compared with the fingers (Fig. 6.8). This orientation is easily seen by the contrasting plane of the thumb by looking at the plane of finger nails. Hence the plane of extension and flexion is across the palm of the hand. Abduction lifts the thumb from the hand and adduction brings the finger into the hand. Thumb flexion and extension are assessed by asking the subject to first flex then extend the thumb to the thenar eminence against resistance. Abduction is assessed by resisting the subject attempting to press the thumb into the palm of the hand. Adduction is assessed by resisted adduction away from the hand. When it is impaired the thumb metacarpal cannot be held against the index so the thumb cannot be held extended when holding

a block in adduction. The thumb will flex at the interphalangeal and metacarpophalangeal joint (Fig. 6.9). Opposition of the thumb is most easily assessed by seeing if an O ring made by the subject by opposing index and thumb can be broken by the observer.

Bunnell's test is important to clarify if resisted flexion is due to contracture or tethering of the intrinsic muscles rather than joint disease. With the metacarpophalangeal joints extended ask the subject to flex the interphalangeal joints. If this is restricted ask the subject to flex the metacarpophalangeal joints. If the flexion at the interphalangeal joints improves there is intrinsic muscle tightness. If there is no change restriction is due to joint disease.

A similar test establishes if restriction of flexion at the proximal interphalangeal joint is due to tendon contracture. If flexion of distal interphalangeal joints is greater when the proximal interphalangeal joints are flexed there is retinacular restriction; if it does not change it is restricted by joint disease.

Nerves

The neurological component of examining the hand is to establish if there is a peripheral neuropathy, a mononeuritis of the radial, median, or the ulnar nerve, or a root lesion involving C6, 7, 8. Skin innervation is C6 on the radial

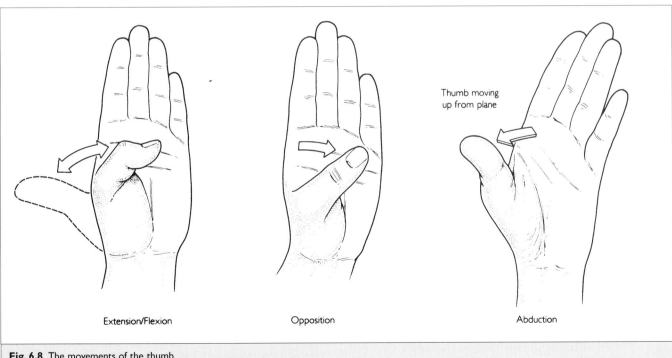

Extension/Flexion   Opposition   Thumb moving up from plane   Abduction

Fig. 6.8 The movements of the thumb.

Weak — Adductor cannot hold metacarpal against index, so thumb cannot be held extended. it flexes at the MCP and ICP

Normal

Fig. 6.9 Testing for thumb adductor weakness.

aspect, C7 on the middle ray and C8 on the medial ulnar aspect. The ulnar nerve sensory supply involves the little and medial half of the ring finger. There is considerable overlap between different people. The radial nerve supplies a variable area of the dorsal aspect of the hand except the distal phalanx. Otherwise the supply is from the medial nerve.

Light touch tested on the radial side of the index, the ulnar side of the little and on the middle finger will establish if there is a neuropathy. If a more proximal neurological abnormality in the cord or brain is suspected then all modalities of sensation including joint position, temperature and pain need to be analysed.

Motor supply is best remembered as a sequence going distally, from wrist extension and flexion—C7, finger flexion and extension—C8, and small muscle of the hand—T1. Wrist extension also takes root supply from C6 and extension from C8. Extension of the wrist and fingers is radial nerve. Flexion and extension of the little and ring finger as well as finger abduction and adduction are ulnar nerve. The medial nerve supplies the inervation for the index, middle and thumb long flexors and a varying supply to the small muscles of the thumb. Only the abductor pollicis brevis of the thenar eminence is reliably supplied by the medial nerve. The ulnar nerve is derived from the median cord of the brachial plexus and C8, T1 roots. The median nerve is

derived from the lateral and median cord and roots C5, 6, 7, 8 and T1. Loss of power is tested by asking the patient to contract a muscle group such as extending the wrist and then the examiner assesses the power needed to overcome the action.

Sensory loss from a peripheral neuropathy gives a characteristic glove pattern of loss. Root lesions may give patchy loss in their anatomical zones. Specific patterns of loss are associated with brachial plexus lesions. Involvement of C6 and 7 gives the Erb palsy pattern. The wrist and fingers are flexed with an extended elbow in the 'waiter's' arm deformity. In paralysis from damage to roots of T1, Kumpje's deformity gives small muscle wasting and clawing of the hand.

The median nerve (Fig 6.10)

The key to establishing if a median nerve lesion is present is if there is sensory loss. Motor involvement is subtle. Assess

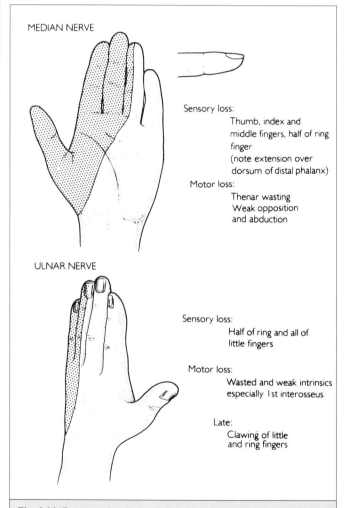

MEDIAN NERVE

Sensory loss:
  Thumb, index and middle fingers, half of ring finger
  (note extension over dorsum of distal phalanx)

Motor loss:
  Thenar wasting
  Weak opposition and abduction

ULNAR NERVE

Sensory loss:
  Half of ring and all of little fingers

Motor loss:
  Wasted and weak intrinsics especially 1st interosseus

Late:
  Clawing of little and ring fingers

Fig. 6.10 Features of median and ulnar nerve lesions.

wasting of the thenar eminence and power of abductor pollicis brevis. This may be difficult in early partial lesions and assessment is often confounded by secondary wasting associated with osteoarthritis of the carpometacaral joint of the thumb. Ask the subject to palmar flex the thumb and hold it against the examiner's resistance. The examiner feels the opponens pollicis, which is the most medial small muscle in the thenar eminence as it contracts. Confirmatory tests, such as Tinel's when the wrist is pressed on in dorsiflexion over the median nerve or Phalen's when the nerve is percussed in the carpal tunnel, have been shown to have very poor sensitivity so give no valuable information. If the clinical signs are not clear a precise diagnosis for a mononeuritis will require electrophysiology.

A proximal lesion of the median nerve above the origin of the anterior interosseous nerve will cause wasting of the long flexors and the index finger will be held extended. The hand is held as if in a benediction attitude.

The radial nerve

The characteristic feature is weak wrist dorsiflexion. If it is mild this may be minimal. More severe lesions and long-standing lesions may give a wrist drop and wasting of muscles in the forearm. Sensory loss is usually minimal because of overlapping supply but may give an area of loss on the dorsum of the hand. If the supinator is involved the lesion must be proximal. Supinator weakness is detected by testing supination of the extended arm at the elbow to reduce the action of the biceps. More proximal lesions cause weakness of the triceps.

The ulna nerve (Fig. 6.10)

The key to identifying an ulnar nerve palsy is wasting and loss of power of the first dorsal interosseous in association with sensory loss to touch in the little and ring finger. Often the ring finger will divide down the middle with loss only on the medial side, in contrast to a root lesion. Wasting and loss of power of the first dorsal interosseous is detected by asking the patient to spread the fingers and maintain abduction of the index finger against resistance as the first dorsal interosseous muscle is palpated with the index finger.

In an established ulnar nerve palsy there will be a contracture of the little and index finger. The metacarpophalangeal joints are extended and the interphalangeal joints

flexed. If the lesion is above the supply to the flexor digitorum profundus, the distal interphalangeal joints will be straight, if below, it will be flexed.

Blood supply

The viability of the circulation is assessed by observing the colour and warmth of the hand, the presence of capillary return and the presence of both ulnar and radial pulses. People vary in the dominance of each artery in supply to the hand. Changes in vessel tone may give Raynaud's and acrocyanosis. Changes in oxygenation will make the fingers cyanosed. The pattern of perfusion can be established by asking the subject to squeeze their hand and the examiner then occluding the ulnar and radial artery with firm finger pressure. The release of pressure on one artery will result in a flush of colour as the perfusion returns.

Longer term ischaemia produces trophic changes. Severe ischaemia will give gangrene and loss of digits. Brachial artery occlusion at the elbow produces a characteristic deformity from muscle contracture due to clawing — Volkmann's contracture (Fig. 6.11). More distal occlusion may give a Bunnell's contracture where the metacarpophalangeal joints are flexed with the fingers extended and the thumb adducted.

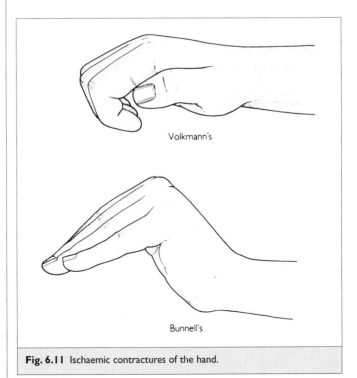

Fig. 6.11 Ischaemic contractures of the hand.

EXAMINATION OF THE ACUTELY TRAUMATISED HAND

Identify key issues needing attention—in particular, is the blood supply endangered? Carefully document lesions and recognise that as the acute problem is addressed other features may become apparent. Repeated assessment is needed.

SCREENING THE HANDS

Look at the resting hands as they rest supinated and pronated. Look proximally to distally. Ask the patient to make a fist with the thumb outside, then make a pinch grip with index and thumb. Feel the pulse and for local tenderness. Test touch sensation on the lateral aspect of the little finger, the radial aspect of the index and the middle finger. Test the power of the first interosseous and the abductor pollicis brevis.

THE HAND IN SYSTEMIC DISEASE

Examination of most 'systems' starts in the hand. There is a need to observe quickly if any clues to key abnormalities are present. In the cardiorespiratory examination, these are is clubbing (Fig. 6.12), cyanosis and splinter haemorrhages. In the abdominal examination these are clubbing and a palmar flush. In thyroid disease it is the development of tremor and acropachy. However, it is in connective tissue disease and arthritis that the hand examination provides the greatest window on the disease process. The pattern of involvement and deformity helps delineate the type of arthritis. The functional problem is important in assessing the possibilities for modifying handicap, and there may be features of systemic involvement of rheumatic disease like vascultis.

SUMMARY

Examination of the hand is a search for information on diagnosis and on functional impairment. The approach needs to tailor to the questions produced in the history.

The hands should be examined together initially by inspection, then palpation and finally more detailed assessment of movement and function. Deliberately looking from the wrist distally trains the eye to explore in a logical way that reflects the hand's functional structure. Usually it is most comfortable to look at the hands supine then ask the patient to pronate them. Feel for tenderness around the joints. Following this the patient makes a fist and grips the thumb and little finger. The sensation needs to be checked for light touch and the pulse noted. The routine is elaborated either as problems are found or depending on the history.

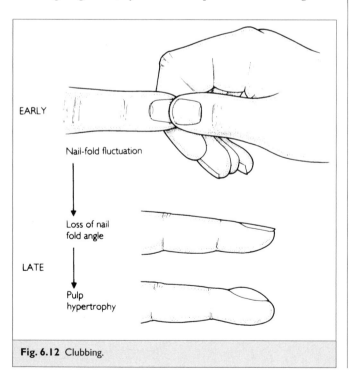

EARLY

Nail-fold fluctuation

Loss of nail fold angle

LATE

Pulp hypertrophy

Fig. 6.12 Clubbing.

7

The spine

Examining the spine seeks to establish if there is a structural problem and if there is abnormal movement. The intimate relationship with the spinal cord and nerve roots and the juxtaposition of the abdomen and chest means information may be needed from a wider neurological examination, including examination of the arms and legs as well as an examination of the chest and abdomen.

PAIN PATTERNS

Spine problems most commonly present with pain. Deformity may develop without symptoms but it is usually pain that makes the patient aware there is a problem. Analysis of the pain pattern is important in identifying likely problems to be explored in the examination. The history provides important leads suggesting if the pain is an intrinsic spinal lesion, if there is referred pain, if the pain is from soft tissue and if it is psychogenic.

The temporal pattern is important. When did it come on? Is it acute, remitting, chronic? Where is it anatomically? Where does it radiate to? What are the associated features, and what worsens or relieves the pain? The character of pain is important in considering the underlying pathology. Inflammatory pain is often worse in the morning and associated with stiffness. Degenerative pain often worsens as the day goes through. Severe unremitting pain suggests malignancy or infection. Pain radiation suggests its origin. Cervical and lumbar pain radiates down the arm or leg. Tenderness associated with pain is an important sign suggesting underlying infection.

Pain of acute onset suggests an acute cause, pain that has gradually developed a more slowly evolving problem. An acute disc prolapse may present with acute pain. Repeated episodes of mechanical pain may evolve into a constant backache. Unremitting severe pain and night pain are sinis-

ter features and suggest underlying malignancy or focal infection. There may be associated features of night sweats and weight loss. Night pain needs to be distinguished from night disturbance as the patient cannot get to sleep because of discomfort.

Pain may be referred to the spine. Abdominal, retroperitoneal and mediastinal structures may give pain referred to the back (Fig. 7.1). Pancreatic and gastric disease may refer to the back so enquiry about other symptoms in the history is important and may heighten the importance of an abdominal or chest examination.

Soft-tissue pain is perhaps the most common type of pain. Its cause and classification continues to be a challenge. Often there is poor correlation of symptoms and signs and it may form a wider pattern. Fibromyalgia gives focal tender points and is associated with fatigue and aches at other sites. Myofascial pain has a characteristic distribution (Fig. 7.2) that can be experimentally mimicked by saline injection into paraspinal structures.

Pain is ultimately a subjective experience. The patient's perception and experience will influence his or her reporting of the symptom. It is influenced by the spinal and cortical

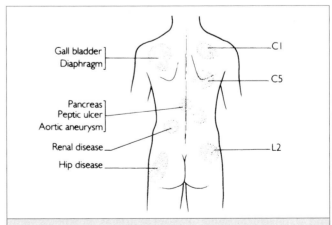

Fig. 7.1 Patterns of referred pain from the viscera to the back.

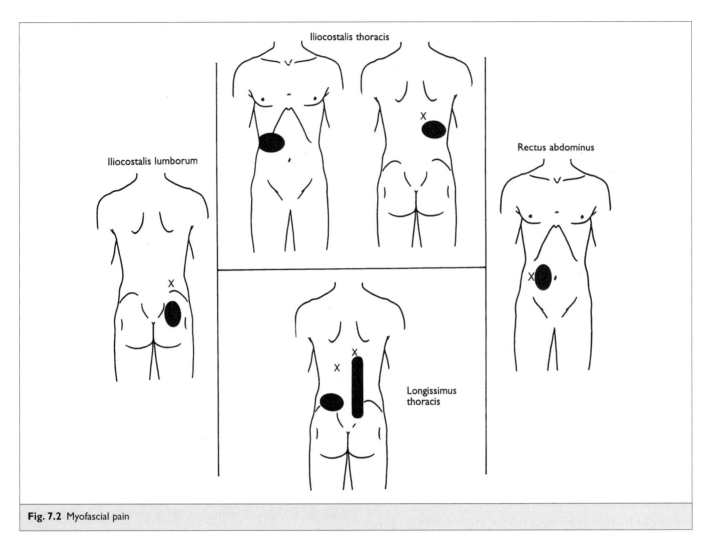

Fig. 7.2 Myofascial pain

processing of information to give patterns that are inconsistent. Debate continues on how much this results in chronic pain—a malfunctioning pain system that results in the persistence of pain unassociated with an initiating pathology. Whether this is a reflection of a psychological reaction, conscious or unconscious, or is malingering is often difficult to analyse. Inconsistency in story and signs is a key to suggesting a psychogenic component to pain.

Pain restricts function. If there is a mechanical problem movement makes it worse. Pain on a constant level of exercise that is relieved by rest may be due to spinal stenosis.

FUNCTIONAL ANATOMY

The spine has several functions. It acts as a scaffold for the abdomen and thorax from which the limbs articulate through the pelvic and shoulder girdle. The rib-cage restricts and stabilises the spine. The spine acts as a crane to allow bending. It is a protective casing for the spinal cord. It sup-

ports the head and allows rotation of the head. The protecting, supporting and moving function means there is a need to provide it with stability and movement.

The basic unit of the spine is the vertebra and disc. The vertebra has a body and posterior arch of pedicle, lamina and transverse and spinous processes. They are arranged in an array. The organisation is best considered as aligned in two columns—the anterior column of vertebral bodies and discs and a posterior column of vertebral arches linked by synovial apophyseal joints. The two columns are linked by pedicles.

The array is held in an oxbow-like curve with cervical and lumbar lordosis and a thoracic kyphosis (Fig. 7.3). There are twelve thoracic, seven cervical, and five lumbar vertebrae. Five sacral vertebrae are fused and there are four vestigial coccygeal vertebrae. Each vertebra and disc can only move a small amount but the net effect of several vertebra moving is to allow considerable movement without reducing stability (Fig. 7.4). The amount of movement in

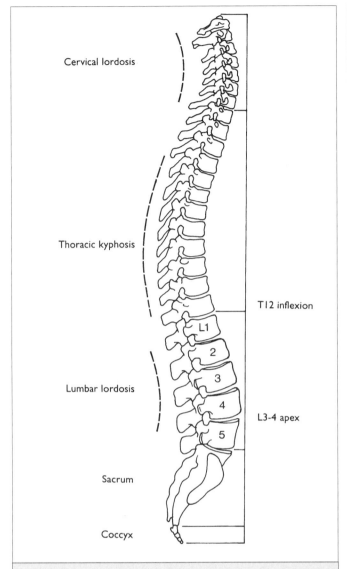

Fig. 7.3 The configuration of the vertebral column.

Cervical lordosis

Thoracic kyphosis

T12 inflexion

L1

2

3

4

5

Lumbar lordosis

L3-4 apex

Sacrum

Coccyx

Fig. 7.4 Lateral flexion. Small amounts of movement between each vertebra can be stabilised and summed to allow large deflections

lateral flexion, flexion extension and rotation varies at different levels of the spine.

Each vertebra has distinct anatomical characteristics (Fig. 7.5). Between each vertebra, except C1 and C2, are discs. These are composed of a central nucleus pulposus, which is a jelly-like material derived from the notocord, and contained by the annulus fibrosus. There are seven cervical vertebrae. The first and second, the atlas and axis, are specialised. C1, the atlas, has no body but an anterior facet joint articulating with the dens. C2, the axis, has the dens projecting superiorly from the vertebral body. The typical cervical vertebra has a spinous process that is bifid, has superior articular facets that articulate backwards and upwards, and a triangular vertebral foramen. C7 has a prominent vertebral spinous process. In the adult skeleton the intervertebral discs do not completely cover the vertebral plate so two synovial oncovertebral joints develop. The posterior wall of the pharynx is close to the anterior column.

The thoracic vertebrae have two pairs of costovertebral facets, and a pair of costal facets on the transverse process; the vertebral foramen is rounded, the spinous processes project inferiorly and the superior articular facets are vertical, flat and face back and laterally. The lumbar vertebrae are large, have no costal facets, a triangular vertebral foramen, the spinous processes project straight back and the superior articular facets orientate backwards and medially. The thoracic spine has restricted mobility compared to the lumbar and cervical spine as it is buttressed by the ribs. Each vertebra has two sets of three articulations with its pair of ribs. Contraction of the extrinsic intercostals raises the ribs in inspiration and the diaphragm contracts to flatten at the same time. The anterior abdominal muscles also contract. In expiration the internal intercostals contract coordinated with contraction of transverse abdominis and thoracis and the subcostal muscles to depress the ribs. Changes in the thoracic spine will produce deformity in the chest wall as it alters the line of orientation of the ribs. It also alters the position of the shoulder and may require compensatory changes in the lumbar and cervical spine.

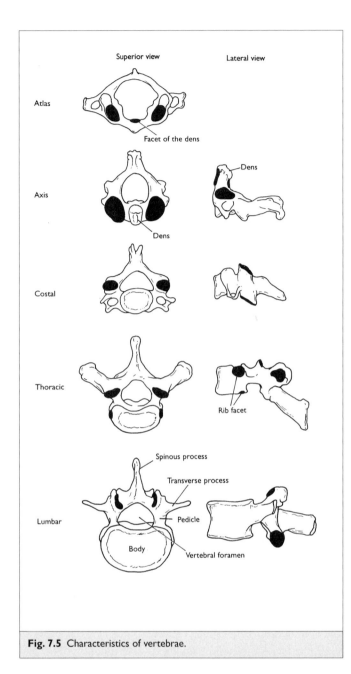

Superior view   Lateral view

Atlas

Facet of the dens

Axis   Dens

Dens

Costal

Thoracic   Rib facet

Spinous process

Transverse process

Lumbar   Pedicle

Body   Vertebral foramen

Fig. 7.5 Characteristics of vertebrae.

There are five lumbar vertebrae, which are held in a lordosis. The first sacral vertebra may be lumbarised with a fully developed disc at S1/S2 or the lumbar vertebra may be sacralised and fused. There are frequent other bone abnormalities or variants with sacralisation of the vertebral process or incomplete fusion of the vertebral arch resulting in spin bifida occulta and poorly developed pars interarticularis in spondylolisthesis. The psoas muscle has its origin on the anterior lumbar spine. An abscess in the psoas muscle will track to the groin. Spasm of the muscle will produce hip flexion.

The orientation of the facets is important in determining the restriction of movement. Little rotation is allowed by the lumbar facets, more rotation is allowed at the thoracic vertebrae and considerable movement is allowed by the flatter cervical facets.

The structure is stabilised by a set of ligaments. On the vertebral body are anterior and posterior longitudinal ligaments. The anterior ligament is attached to the disc and body with a potential space where osteophytes develop as degenerative change occurs. The posterior longitudinal ligament is only attached to the disc and a potential space behind the body is filled by the paravertebral venous plexus. In the vertebral foramen the ligamentum flavum links the lamina of the posterior arch and the capsular ligaments of the apophyseal joints. There are a set of ligaments linking the transverse and spinous processes. The intertransverse ligament is prominent in the lumbar spine. The supraspinous ligament is prominent in the neck and joins the tips of the spinous processes as the ligamentum nuchae. There is an interspinous ligament and anterior and posterior articular process ligaments associated with the capsular ligaments. A complex set of ligaments link the lumbar spine to the pelvis. There are iliolumbar ligaments linking the transverse processes of L4 to the superior iliac crest and from L5 to the superior and inferior iliac crest as well as the sacrum. A set of ligaments—the sacroiliac ligament, sacrospinous ligament and sacrotuberous ligament—link to the ischial spine, sacral spinous processes and ischial tuberosity, as well as the anterior and inferior sacroiliac ligaments that cross the sacroiliac joints anteriorly.

The arterial supply is from the arteries that in turn are branches of the subclavian vertebral, deep cervical, intervertebral and lumbar arteries. Anterior and posterior radicular arteries form the anterior spinal artery of the cord and this supplies all except the posterior columns of the cord, which are supplied by the posterior spinal artery. The lower two-thirds of the spine may be supplied by one large artery, the radicularis magna artery of Adamkiewicz. The venous drainage is via a plexus of veins that drain to the cavae and azygos vein.

The spinal cord ends at the body of L2 and a leash of nerve roots run down the canal as the cauda equina. For each segment of the cord paired superior dorsal and ventral roots fuse to give the nerve root that exits through the vertebral foramen. This is in close to the apophyseal joint and in the cervical spine to the vertebral artery and neurocentral joints. The root then divides into anterior and posterior primary rami (Fig. 7.6).

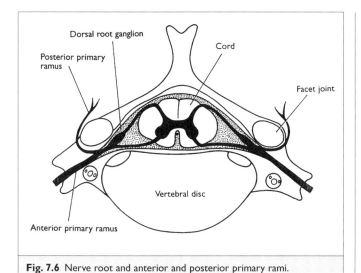

Fig. 7.6 Nerve root and anterior and posterior primary rami.

The vertebral canal is narrower at the root of the neck and widens superiorly. The cord is expanded in the lower section. A canal with a sagittal diameter of less than 13 mm will be vulnerable to compression. The normal sagittal diameter is 15–20 mm. The cord is elastic. In flexion the cord stretches some 2 cm and it tends to buckle in extension. The movement is limited by nerve roots and the ligamentum denticulatum laterally. The roots emerge through intervetebral foramina superior to their vertebral bodies. So, for example, the C6 root emerges above the body of C6 and is approximately at the level of the C5/6 disc. The dura folds as the neck extends.

The spinal structures are innervated by the sinuvertebral nerves. Their irritation causes sclerotomal referral. The level of referral, however, may alter as the spine changes configuration with loss of disc height. The superficial layer of the annulus fibrosus is innervated but probably not the more central disc tissue.

The segmental organisation of the cord means that each root supplies a defined dermatome, sclerotome and myotome. The sensation loss or symptoms affecting a root may be referred in a dermatomal distribution (Fig. 7.7). The cervical dermatome distribution is indistinct with considerable overlap, so gives poor localising information. However, C2 supplies an area of the angle of the jaw and lobe of the ear that is helpful in deciding if facial loss is or is not hysterical or malingering. In the lumbar and cervical spine myotome information from loss of muscle power or reflex loss is more precise (Table 7.1). The approximate sensory levels in the thoracic spine are given by the nipple line at T5, and the umbilicus at T10.

MOVEMENT

In the cervical spine the muscles that move the neck are arranged in layers. There is a superficial layer of trapezius and sternocleidomastoid, and a deep band of intrinsic muscles linking the spinal process of the vertebra that allow movement in flexion, extension anterioposteriorly, flexion laterally and rotation. To achieve rotation an element of

Table 7.1 Root lesions

	Sensory loss (supply)	Area of pain	Reflex loss	Motor deficit
L2	Often none (upper upper thigh)	Across thigh	None	Hip flexion
L3	Often none (across lower thigh)	Across thigh	Adductor	Knee flexion
L4	Medial leg (across knee to medial malleolus)	Down to medial malleolus	Knee	Inversion of foot
L5	Dorsum of foot (side of leg to dorsum of foot)	Back of thigh, calf, dorsum of foot	None	Dorsiflexion of toes and of foot (with L4)
S1	Behind lateral malleolus (behind lateral malleolus to lateral foot	Back of thigh, calf, lateral foot	Ankle jerk	Plantar flexion and eversion of foot
C5	Lateral border of arm (lateral border of arm)	Lateral border of arm	Biceps	Deltoid infra- and supraspinatus
C6	Lateral border of forearm and thumb (lateral border of forearm and thumb)	Lateral border of forearm	Supinator	Biceps pronator and supinator of forearm
C7	Middle fingers (middle forearm and middle finger	Middle fingers	Triceps	Wrist extensors and flexors triceps
C8	Medical forearm and little finger (medial forearm and little finger)	Medial forearm and little finger	Finger jerk	Finger flexors, extensors
T1	Axilla (axilla)	Axilla	None	Small muscles of the hand

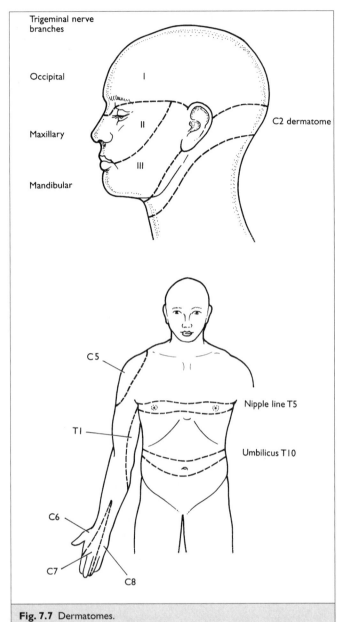

Fig. 7.7 Dermatomes.

the young the spine may be very mobile. The muscles that produce a given movement vary depending on whether the spine is vertical or supine. Analysis provides little anatomical localising information except that the trapezius is innervated along with sternocleidomastoid by the 11th cranial nerve. Flexion of the spine involves longissimus cervicis, scaleni, semispinalis and rectus abdominis; extension involves erector spinae, splenius and semispinalis; lateral flexion uses longissimus, iliocostalis cervicis and the obliques; finally rotation involves the rotatores, multifidus and splenius cervicis.

EXAMINATION

The spine may be considered as one unit, or examined in each of the components—cervical, thoracic and lumbar spine—to allow a logical process of examination for the particular problem identified in the history and to suit the comfort of the patient. The approach is to observe, assess movement, palpate—look, move, feel. Most is learned from observation. This starts as the patient comes into the room. Watch their posture and gait, watch them undress, and then look formally with the patient undressed to underclothes. Remember that examination of the chest, abdomen and hips, as well as assessment of neurological signs, may be needed to complete the clinical examination.

The cervical spine

Look

Observe the subject come into the room. Do they hold their neck normally or is it held rigidly? As they undress is the neck flexed and extended to remove items of clothing? Formal examination is best done with the patient lying supine to relax the muscles of the neck. Then examine the patient either standing or sitting to assess posture and movement.

Examining the cervical spine is part of the examination of the neck. The neck has three zones to assess: anterior, lateral and posterior (Fig. 7.8). The sternomastoid crosses diagonally from the occiput to the sternoclavicular joint and delineates a boundary of the anterior neck and lateral triangle. The third zone is the back of the neck observed from behind and is delineated by the trapezius muscle.

Anteriorly identify and palpate the midline structures: the hyoid bone, the laryngeal prominence or Adam's apple, the cricoid cartilage, the thyroid and the trachea descending

lateral flexion is needed. The atlanto-axial, and atlanto-occipital section of the spine is particularly mobile. In the upper cervical spine the atlanto-occipital joint accounts for about 20° flexion and 5° of lateral flexion. The movement in nodding largely occurs at this joint. Rotation is minimal. At the atlanto-axial joint most rotation is allowed. There is 15° of rotation to each side, which needs some lateral flexion and extension to slacken the alar ligaments. In the lower cervical spine flexion/extension of 110° is possible. From neutral there is about 85° of flexion and 15° of extension; 40° of lateral flexion and axial rotation of 50° to each side is possible.

With age there is a gradual reduction in movement and in

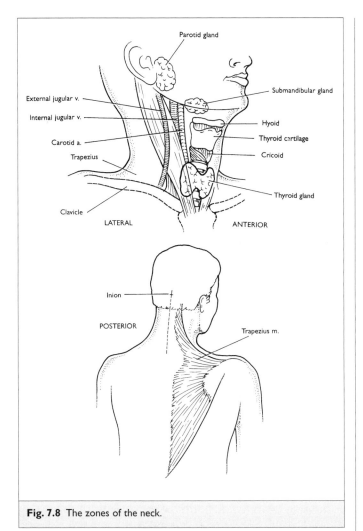

Fig. 7.8 The zones of the neck.

Fig. 7.9 Palpating the neck.

into the jugular notch. The transverse process of the atlas is at the level of the lateral end of the hyoid bone and can be felt as the neck rotates. The thyroid can be felt more easily if the patient is asked to take a sip of water and swallow it as the examiner gently palpates the neck. It may be easier to assess feeling round the neck from behind when the patient is sitting (Fig. 7.9). The thyroid lies as an H shape soft-tissue swelling across the trachea at the level of C4. The hyoid bone is at the level of C3 and like the thyroid moves with swallowing. The 1st cricoid cartilage ring is at the level of the body of C6. Lateral to this is the bony prominence of the carotid tubercle (Fig. 7.10).

Assess the body of the sternomastoid and note its insertions into the clavicle and sternum. Note if the sternoclavicular joint is prominent or tender. Note the curve of the clavicle. Bony deformity may persist from fracture and the bone may be diffusely enlarged by Paget's disease. Feel in the supra- and infraclavicular fossa for nodes. In the anterior angle of the lateral triangle made by the clavicle and the ster-

Fig. 7.10 The position of the hyoid bone, thyroid and 1st cricoid cartilage.

nomastoid, the body of the omohyoid can be felt, the pulse of the subclavian may be felt and a cervical rib may be noted. The pulsation in the external jugular vein can be seen and the pulsation of the carotid felt below the angle of the jaw. The parotid gland is felt just superior to the line of the jaw and the submandibular gland under the mandible. The mastoid can be felt behind the ear and just anterior of the mastoid is the styloid process. Lymph nodes may be present along the edge of the sternomastoid. Ask the patient to grimace to make the platysma muscle prominent.

It may be necessary to examine the ear, temporomandibular joint, oropharynx and chest.

Observe the neck with the patient sitting or standing, anteriorly, laterally and posteriorly. Is the posture correct with a straight spine in the sagittal line and a normal curve seen laterally? Anterior examination will establish if the neck is held straight—with level shoulders and level eyes. If not there may be a torticollis. Then examination needs to establish if problems with the lower spine are being compensated in the neck. If a torticollis develops before growth has stopped facial asymmetry may develop. Laterally observe the contour of the neck and how this relates to a thoracic kyphosis. Posteriorly look for the spinous processes of T1 and C7.

A short rigid neck may be associated with developmental problems such as juvenile chronic arthritis or Klippel–Feil syndrome; a webbed neck is associated with Turner's syndrome. In infancy torticollis is associated with a sternocleidomastoid tumour. In adults it may result from disc disease or strabismus.

Feel

Palpate for tenderness. Marked focal tenderness needs explaining as there is a possibility of underlying infection. Reactive nodes may be tender. Muscles, particularly the trapezius, may be focally tender and have increased tone, so seem knotted in response to pain or as part of a fibromyalgia or a myofascial pain problem. Lymph nodes can be palpated along the sternocleidomastoid, the nuchal line and in the supraclavicular fossa. The submandibular glands and parotids should be felt. The thyroid should be examined. It is easier to identify if the patient takes a small drop of water and swallows it whilst the gland is gently palpated and can be felt to move. Warn the patient what needs to be done and that he or she is not being strangled. The carotid pulses should be felt and if there is a history of vascular disease or strokes the patient should be auscultated for bruits.

Posteriorly the line of the neck is centred on the inion in the centre of the nuchal line. The spinous process can be felt below this with the most prominent, the vertebra prominens

of C7. The trapezius originates from these processes and runs down to insert in a fan on the spine of the scapula and the chest wall. Embryonically it is derived from the same muscle as sternocleidomastoid and shares 11th nerve innervation.

Move

This is best done with the patient seated or standing. If a measure of movement is needed ask the patient to hold a rod in the mouth to accentuate the angle (Fig. 7.11). As a rule of thumb, in full extension the tip of the nose and forehead should form a horizontal line and the occiput will be at the level of the spinous process of T1. Anterior flexion should allow the chin to touch the chest wall. If it cannot, one finger or more can be put between the chin and chest wall to estimate the loss. One finger means that about 10° of movement has been lost. In rotation the chin should turn almost to the shoulder in the coronal plane. Rotation largely occurs at the altanto-axial joint, nodding at the altanto-occipital joint and flexion and extension in the mid-cervical spine.

Watch the subject move first. Explain carefully what is needed. In lateral flexion people will usually move their shoulder up to their ear so gentle restraint on the shoulder will remind them to flex the neck laterally. Is motion smooth and not in pain or is it jerky and restricted? Check the range of passive movement. If the head is gently held during movement then at any limit the examiner can gently explore if the range can be increased passively. This should not be done if there is a risk that the cervical cord is damaged or the neck is unstable, for example after trauma. It is usually possible to see what a particular range of active movement is and then see if increased passive range can be demonstrated by gently pushing the range further.

The only individual muscles to check are the sternocleidomastoid and trapezius to confirm nerve supply by the accessory, 11th cranial nerve. The trapezius is tested by asking the patient to shrug and then repeat this against resistance. The sternocleidomastoid is tested by asking the subject to rotate the neck against the resistance of the examiner's hand on the jaw. The examiner palpates the contracting muscle with the other hand. The net strength of the flexors is tested simply by asking the patient to put his or her chin on the chest when lying and resisting the examiner trying to extend the neck. Similarly, the examiner holds a hand on the occiput to resist extension and obtain a net assessment of extensor power. For lateral flexion and rotation a similar

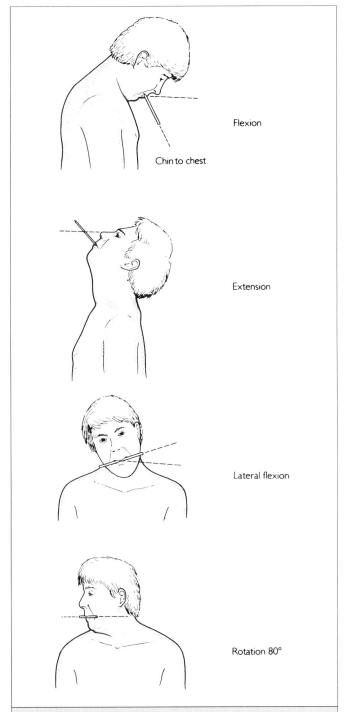

Flexion

Chin to chest

Extension

Lateral flexion

Rotation 80°

Fig. 7.11 Assessing movement of the neck. A pencil held by the subject's mouth allows more accurate assessment of loss.

Barber chair sign, (Lhermitte's sign). Flexion of the neck may produce paraesthesia down the arms or legs in multiple sclerosis or spondylosis.

Spurling's manoeuvre. Downward pressure on the neck may induce symptoms from vertebral foramina narrowing. This can be accentuated by pressing during lateral flexion. Root symptoms may be induced if held for 10 seconds. If there is a risk of malignancy, infection, odontoid disease or fracture this should not be done. Conversely, cervical traction by pulling the occiput and jaw up may relieve root entrapment symptoms.

Foraminal compression test. Press down on the head to 'compress' the cervical spine. Pain in a vulnerable root may be induced.

Valsalva manoeuvre. Holding the breath against a closed glottis or coughing increases the intrathecal pressure and may induce pain from a tumour or disc prolapse.

Thoracic outlet signs—Adson's manoeuvre. There is considerable controversy over clinical examination to identify signs confirming thoracic outlet problems. They have poor sensitivity and specificity. Adson's manoeuvre involves further constricting the subclavian arterial flow and pulse. If the subclavian artery is being compromised there may be a bruit. If the arm is raised, extended and externally rotated, then the head is rotated to the arm and the radial pulse felt and a bruit listened for over the subclavian. Pulling the arm down may also reduce the brachial pulse and induce T1 symptoms. Abducting the arm above the level of the shoulder will, however, often abolish the radial pulse in normal subjects.

Localisation of a neurological abnormality in the neck requires a careful neurological examination. Common problems are root entrapment, cervical myelopathy or a risk of instability at the atlanto-axial junction. With root entrapment, symptoms localise poorly to the dermatome. Reflex loss and distal upper motor signs of increased tone and increased reflexes may be helpful in localising the level (Fig. 7.11). Cervical myelopathy presents primarily with upper motor neuron problems in the legs so disease of the spinal cord will require a detailed neurological examination. Sympathetic trunk damage may produce an autonomic lesion and cause Horner's syndrome.

manoeuvre of resisted movement is all that can be done. Often it is sensible to hold the patient's shoulder with the free hand. For rotation hold the mandible to resist rotation while the other hand steadies the shoulder. A screen to test for fatigue of neck muscles is to ask the patient to hold the neck flexed for a minute when lying supine.

Thoracic spine

Look

Look from behind with the subject standing. Is the spine straight? Imagine a plumb line hanging from the vertebra prominens of C7. There is often a slight scoliosis and associated rotation of the spine in normal people. A prominent scoliosis needs to be assessed (Fig. 7.12).

First, see if it is compensatory. That is, can it be corrected by correcting a leg length inequality? If it can, it should be abolished by sitting. If not, it is fixed or positional. If when the patient bends forward and the curve disappears the spine is mobile, the curve is probably positional. If it persists, it is structural. Bending may make it more prominent. Scoliosis is associated with a rotation of the vertebrae so the ribs are abnormally aligned. The result is that the ribs push up out of the concavity, so as the patient goes forward a prominent distortion of the posterior chest wall is seen. A curve is usually compensated by other curves above and/or below. These initially are mobile but may over time become fixed. The curves may increase with an individual's growth.

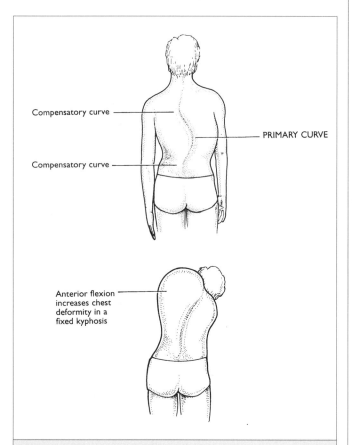

Compensatory curve

PRIMARY CURVE

Compensatory curve

Anterior flexion increases chest deformity in a fixed kyphosis

Fig. 7.12 A thoracolumbar scoliosis.

The primary curve is described to specify if the scoliosis is convex to the left or right.

The side designated by the convexity designates the type of curve, left or right. A right scoliosis has a curve that is convex to the right. Commonly, scoliosis is idiopathic but it may complicate neurological disease such as polio and neurofibromatosis, syringomyelia and myopathies. Degenerative disc disease is often associated with a moderate scoliosis. It may result from focal neoplasm or infection. These are often painful and a painful scoliosis needs investigation and a detailed examination of the neurological system is needed to assess if there is associated muscle or spinal cord disease such as syringomyelia.

There are five patterns of idiopathic scolioses. In infants a convex curve to the left is commoner in males (60%). In adolescents 90% occur in females and 90% are convex to the right; half progress to a severe kyphosis. A thoracolumbar scoliosis is more common in females and is slightly more commonly convex to the right. A lumbar scoliosis is equally left or right and is more common in females. It is often missed until it becomes symptomatic later in life. Thoracic and lumbar scolioses may combine and produce compensatory curves and little deformity.

Look from the side. Look at the thoracic kyphosis to see if the outline is altered. There may be a sudden increase as in curve from a gibbus, or a general increase in the angle of the curve (Fig. 7.13). The former occurs with infective discitis, the later with disc degenerative disease, multiple wedge fracture, disc disease, muscle disease and idiopathic senile kyphosis. In adolescents there may be an increase in kyphosis from Scheuermann's disease. A kyphosis will give abdominal cramping and a protuberant abdomen. The associated loss of height may result in the lower ribs impinging on the iliac blade and cause fat and skin folds in the loin and across the back.

Move

Movement of the thoracic spine is restricted by the ribs. Flexion, extension and lateral flexion and extension are assessed by measuring the distance from the processes of T1 to T12. Anterior flexion increases this by 3 cm and allows 45° of bend: 20° of extension is normal. Lateral flexion is assessed from behind, watching the patient run an arm down the lateral aspect of the leg towards the knee, allowing 15° of bend. Flexion, extension and lateral flexion are all integrated with lumbar movement. Rotation is assessed by asking the

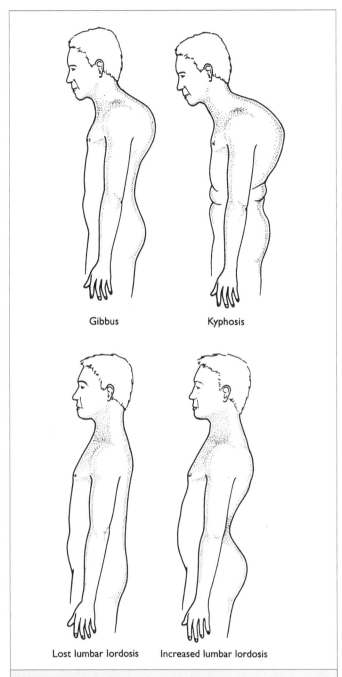

Gibbus

Kyphosis

Lost lumbar lordosis

Increased lumbar lordosis

Fig. 7.13 Lateral inspection of the thoracolumbar spine to show an acute kyphosis or gibbus, lost or increased lumbar lordosis.

patient to sit. This enables the examiner to make sure the pelvis is fixed. The patient then turns to look over the shoulder. Fifteen degrees of thoracic rotation and 5° of lumbar rotation are generated by a combination of both sections of the spine. Movement of the costovertebral joints is assessed by chest expansion, which should be 5 cm at the nipple line.

Feel

Focal tenderness of the thoracic spine can be assessed by gently percussing the spine. Localised tenderness needs careful assessment. Examine for tenderness in the renal angle and to assess rib encroachment on the iliac blade. Feel for spasm in the paravertebral muscles. Note if there are knots of tender muscle or points triggering tenderness. Referred pain may be associated with 'tenderness'. Muscle pain may be referred in rather unusual patterns determined by myotome.

The lumbar spine

The lumbar spine is held in a lordosis. Disease may result in a loss of the lordotic curve and loss of movement. Changes in the spine may cause root entrapment so neurological examination may be necessary. Neurological disease in the cord that stops at L2 and corda equina must be considered and a careful neurological examination may be needed. Look especially for saddle sensory loss.

Symptoms from the lumbar spine are often referred from the abdomen. This must also be examined, with rectal and vaginal examination as appropriate. Blood pressure and urine analysis will help identify possible renal causes. Symptoms in the lumbar spine may originate from the sacroiliac joints and hips, which should be assessed as part of the examination. Pain from the spine may be referred into the legs and present as hip or even knee problems. Claudication may be due to either peripheral vascular disease or more rarely spinal stenosis when leg pulses will be normal. It is important also to examine the hips, inguinal canal and the abdomen. A psoas abscess will 'point' in the groin and has tracked from the psoas origin on the lumbar spine.

Look

Look from behind and the side, with the patient standing undressed to underclothes. Is the spine straight and the shape of the lordosis normal? There may be a transverse lumbar crease and palpable step suggests there may be a spondylolisthesis. There may be a loss of height with crowding of the ribs, with the lowest ribs touching the iliac crests as a result of loss of the vertebral body height in osteoporosis.

Move (Fig. 7.14)

Ask the subject to bend to extend the spine and then flex forward. Then ask them to flex laterally, running a hand down to the knee. Watch the character of movement. Is it laboured? Is there an element of inconsistency? Is the amount the subject bends less than would be expected from just observing them undress and move around the room? Can the subject extend the spine? The lordosis may increase in pregnancy, flexion deformity of the hips and knees and poor posture. It is lost with muscle spasm that may be associated with disc prolapse and chronic mechanical back pain. It is reduced in inflammatory spine disease such as ankylosing spondylitis. If the spine is fixed, flexion can occur at the hip. This can be noted by measuring the excursion of the lumbar segments and by noting if the normal lumbar lordotic curve is reversed as in normal flexion. If the straight spine or lumbar curve persists, it suggests that the spine is fixed with

Fig. 7.14 Lumbar movement.

most flexion at the hip (Fig. 7.15). Measure the amount of movement by marking identifiable spinous processes such as the spine of T12 and the sacral margin. Anterior flexion should be more than 7 cm. Measurement can also be documented as finger tip distance to the floor or knee at full anterior flexion. The distance from the tips of the fingers to the floor when someone is bending forward is less than 10 cm in the normal subject. Hip flexion can compensate for spinal restriction. Increased spinal movement with extension over 30° and flexion to allow the hands to be placed in dorsiflexion flat on the floor is a feature of hypermobility. Lateral flexion is about 15° and rotation is minimal at 5°. It cannot be delineated from thoracolumbar rotation.

Feel

Feel the spinous processes. Is there a notch that may correspond to a spondylolisthesis? Percuss for local tenderness.

Normal

Stiff spine fails to reverse lordosis in flexion

Hypermobility of the spine

Marked extension

Hands flat on floor

Fig. 7.15 A fixed spine (top) and hypermobile spine (bottom).

Root entrapment

The pattern of pain is important to localising a spinal lesion. Reflex loss and wasting of muscle provides objective pointers in addition to patterns of sensory loss. S1 root lesions may result in loss of the ankle jerk, with soleus wasting. L5 lesions give loss of the dorsiflexor of the great toe with weakness of extensor hallucis longus. Loss of the knee reflex and quadriceps wasting suggests an L4 root lesion. Compare each leg to increase the awareness of differences suggesting diminished reflexes, increased weakness and wasting. Observe the patient lying supine and measure mid-thigh and mid-calf diameter to compare each side. Remember, there may be some inequality related to which leg is dominant. Gastrosoleal wasting and weakness can be very subtle. Pain due to root lesions is supported by using tests that stress the roots. Similarly, non-organic pain may be suggested by seeing if tests that should be negative give pain and if there is inconsistency.

Root stretching tests (Fig. 7.16)

Femoral stretch test. The femoral nerve has roots from L2, 3, 4. The patient lies prone. Passive extension of the hip or flexion of the knee will increase pain.

Sciatic stretch tests. The sciatic nerve roots are L4, 5, S1, 2, 3. With the patient supine flex the hip with the knee extended. This should be possible to 90°. If it is limited assess dorsiflexion of the ankle; pressure behind the knee is possible at the limit of straight leg raising. It should increase pain as they further increase the sciatic root. With the knee flexed, flex the hip and then straighten the knee to see if the limit to straight leg raising is consistent.

Contralateral straight leg raising test. Raise the contralateral leg and observe if pain induced in the symptomatic leg. It is considered to have greater sensitivity for a root lesion.

Tests suggesting malingering

Passive extension test. The patient lies supine with the hip and knees flexed and supported by the examiner. The examiner lowers the uninvolved side and confirms there is no pain. The involved side is then lowered and the spine extends to give pain. The unaffected leg is then flexed to relieve pain if the pain is organic.

Fig. 7.16 Root stretching tests.

Active flexion test. Ask the patient to lie supine and rest their heels in the examiner's hands. Ask them to lift the affected leg. If they are unable to raise the leg establish if they are pressing down on the contralateral hand. If they are genuinely attempting to lift the leg they should be. Note if agonists and antagonists, such as quadriceps and hamstrings, in the affected leg are being contracted simultaneously, this suggests malingering.

Observe the patient sit up after being examined. They should flex the knee to allow spinal flexion if there is a root problem. Are they inconsistent as they dress? Is pain increased when pressure is applied to the head or shoulders when standing? It should not be if a root lesion is present but an exaggerated response is often seen if the problem is

functional. Can the patient rotate the shoulders forward when standing with arms free? This is primarily thoracolumbar rotation. Is there is no difference if the patient holds their hands on the hips when movement will be predominantly in the legs, it suggests the problem is functional.

Ask the patient to sit after assessing the amount of straight leg raising tolerated when supine. Extend the knee and observe if the patient sits back to reduce sciatic stretch and when the stretch is unacceptable in comparison to when tested supine. Note if a tendency to a scoliosis is maintained if the subject is sitting compared to standing.

The cord ends at L2. Central disc lesions above this will give a cord lesion with upper motor nerve signs; below gives lower motor nerve lesions. There will be multiple root involvement. Two patterns are possible. A high lateral lesion will give multiple root signs. A midline conus lesion may only produce motor problems in S1 and late after saddle analgesia has developed (Fig. 7.17).

The coccyx

This is the vestigial tail. There are usually four segments. Ask the patient to lie on their side and examine the natal cleft. This is a common site for psoriasis. Palpate the coccyx for tenderness. Then examine per rectum, palpating the coccyx anteriorly.

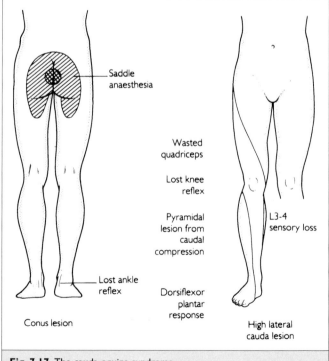

Fig. 7.17 The cauda equina syndrome.

The sacroiliac joints

These are deep structures that are difficult to assess clinically. Observation may show little. Movement is minimal. It may be helpful to try to localise pain to the sacroiliac joints by stressing the joint. There may be focal tenderness, which is important to follow-up. There are two stress tests of the sacroiliac joints (Fig. 7.18). Compress the pelvis by pushing on both iliac blades, or by fixing the pelvis and pushing the contralateral leg flexed at the knee and hip to the patient's contralateral iliac fossa. The sensitivity and specificity of these tests may be poor for eliciting true sacroiliac pain.

SUMMARY

The examination of the spine looks for signs to help clarify the problems that have been identified in the history. The signs may give an indication of the underlying pathology and site. The latter involves careful neurological examination. Because of the proximity and the segmental innervation of the body, problems in the neck, chest and abdomen are often referred to the spine. Consideration of more extensive examination is important. The neck, thoracic spine and lumbar spine are often examined separately.

A QUICK SCREEN EXAMINING THE SPINE

Often a patient is being examined for a problem unrelated to the musculoskeletal system and it is only important to check quickly that there are no other unexpected problems. Look at the patient undressed standing from behind and the side. Ask the patient to move the head to check the cervical spine by looking up, down and laterally flexed right and left. Ask the patient to touch the toes with straight legs. If there are no clear abnormalities it will be unnecessary to examine further.

Compression with 'springing' of the pelvis

Hip flexion and adduction to push knee at contralateral superior iliac blade

Fig. 7.18 Sacroiliac examination.

8

The hip

The hip is a synovium-lined ball-and-socket joint that combines an extensive range of movement with great stability. The stability is due to the relatively deep insertion of the femoral head into the acetabulum and the strong capsule and muscles that surround the joint. The hip plays a major role in weight-bearing and locomotion, so that disorders of the hip are translated quickly into pain and limp. Disordered hip function also disturbs sexual activity.

DEVELOPMENT

The lower limb buds appear at approximately 4 weeks of embryonic life as small lateral outgrowths of the trunk opposite the lumbar and upper sacral segments. At birth, the acetabulum is entirely cartilaginous and sited at the meeting point of the ilium, pubis and ischium which, at this stage of development, are the three separate centres making up the hemipelvis. The centre of ossification in the head of the femur is visible on X-ray at 6 months, while the centre of ossification appears in the greater trochanter at approximately 7 years of age. In adolescence, the head of the femur is well-developed and three epiphyseal lines can be seen: between the head and neck of the femur and outlining the greater and lesser trochanters. These begin to fuse shortly after puberty and fusion is usually complete by the age of 20 years.

Developmental abnormalities

Congenital dislocation of the hip affects approximately one in 1000 babies. One or both hips may be dislocated at birth or dislocate in the first few weeks of life. Girls are affected more than boys and there is a familial tendency. All neonates should be routinely examined for this. The condition can be detected by flexing the hips and knees (Fig. 8.1) and abducting the hips. Normally, the thigh will touch or nearly touch

Fig. 8.1 Examination for congenital dislocation of the hip.

the examining couch. If there is subluxation of the hip, abduction will be limited. The femoral head may be felt slipping into the acetabulum, sometimes with an audible click.

The blood supply to the epiphysis of the head of the femur is vulnerable between the ages of 5 and 10 years. In Perthes' disease, blood supply is impaired, leading to osteonecrosis of the capital epiphysis and resulting in a flattened, misshapen head of the femur.

Slipped femoral epiphysis is a disorder of adolescence affecting boys more than girls. The head of the femur slips inferiorly and posteriorly on the neck, leading to a coxa vara deformity of the hip. This can occur acutely or, more commonly, as a subacute process. Sometimes there is a history of trauma, but mostly the cause is unknown.

Contraction of the iliotibial band can result in a deformity consisting of flexion, abduction and external rotation of the hip, unequal leg length, pelvic tilt and exaggerated lumbar lordosis, valgus deformity and flexion contracture of the knee, external torsion of the tibia on the femur and a secondary equinovarus deformity of the foot. Partial forms of this are most commonly encountered and it is an important cause, for example, of knee pain and ill-defined leg symptoms.

ANATOMY

The proximal part of the femur (Fig. 8.2) consists of the head, neck and greater and lesser trochanters, which are joined by the intertrochanteric line. The head articulates in the acetabular cavity, which is deepened by the glenoid labrum, a circular fibrocartilaginous rim that forms a tight collar around the head of the femur. A gap in the lower portion of the labrum, the acetabular notch, is bridged by the transverse ligament, beneath which blood vessels pass into the joint. The articular cartilage of the acetabulum is horseshoe-shaped and a mass of fat lies in the fossa at the bottom of the acetabulum. The head of the femur is lined with hyaline cartilage. This varies in thickness from about 3 mm at its thickest over the superior and posterior aspects, to about 2 mm at the lateral margin.

There is a strong, dense fibrous capsule. This is attached proximally to the acetabulum, the glenoid facet and the transverse ligament. Distally, it covers the lateral margin of the femoral head and most of the neck. Anteriorly, it is attached to the intertrochanteric line and posteriorly to the neck just above this (Fig. 8.2). The capsule is reinforced in front by the iliofemoral ligament, inferiorly by the pubofemoral ligament and behind by the ischiofemoral ligament.

The ligamentum teres is an intracapsular ligament which arises from the transverse ligament of the acetabular rim,

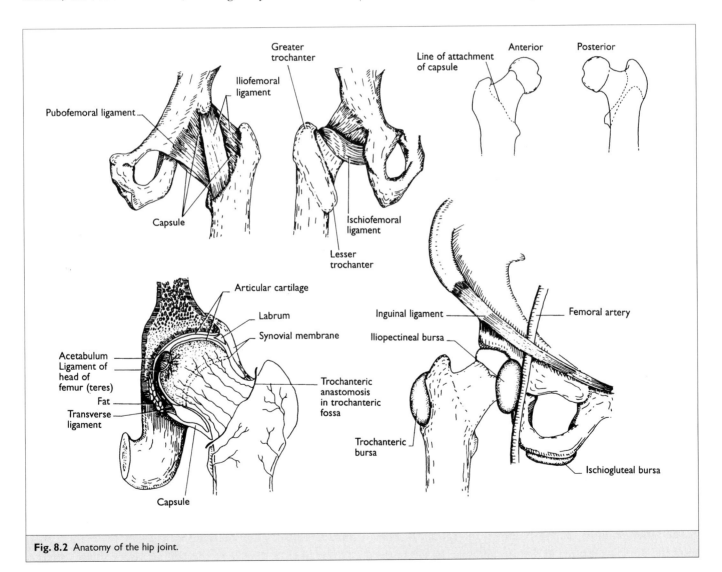

Fig. 8.2 Anatomy of the hip joint.

attaching to a pit in the head of the femur, and carries blood vessels which provide nourishment for a small area of the head adjacent to the attachment of the ligament. On the inner aspect of the distal part of the capsule, fibrous bands carry blood vessels to foramina of the neck and femoral head.

The iliotibial band is a portion of the fascia lata. It extends down the lateral thigh from its major attachment at the iliac crest to the lateral tibial tubercle.

The synovial membrane lines the inner surface of the articular capsule. It covers the glenoid labrum and the mass of fat in the bottom of the acetabular cavity. It also encloses the ligamentum teres. Distally, it is reflected onto the femoral neck and extends to the articular cartilage of the head (Fig. 8.2).

Many bursae have been identified. Those most involved clinically are the iliopectineal (or iliopsoas) bursa, the trochanteric bursa and the ischiogluteal bursa. The iliopectineal bursa lies over the anterior surface of the articular capsule beneath the deep surface of the iliopsoas muscle and between the iliofemoral and pubofemoral ligaments. It is the largest and most constant of the bursae and communicates with the hip joint in approximately 15%. The trochanteric bursa is multilocular and situated between the posterolateral surface of the greater trochanter and the gluteus maximus muscle. It actually comprises three bursae, the principal being the gluteus maximus bursa; the bursae of gluteus medius and gluteus maximus are at the sites of the respective tendon attachments. The ischiogluteal bursa is over the ischial tuberosity and overlies the sciatic nerve. It facilitates gliding of the gluteus maximus over the tuberosity.

The hip joint is surrounded by powerful muscle groups which maintain the upright position of the trunk and assist locomotion. They are summarised in Table 8.1.

SYMPTOMS

Pain is the most common complaint although some severe disorders of the hip, such as congenital dislocation and congenital coxa vara, are typically painless. Limping and other functional deficiencies can be a major feature whether or not the hip is painful. Common disabilities are difficulty getting out of bed in the morning, reaching to put on socks, climbing stairs and sexual intercourse.

The innervation of the leg is shown in Figure 8.3. Pain from the hip joint is often ill-defined and may be felt in the

Table 8.1.   Muscle groups of the hip joint

Movement	Muscle group	Nerve root supply
Flexion		
Prime	Iliopsoas	
Accessory	Rectus femoris	
	Pectineus	L2, 3
	Sartorius	
	Adductor longus	
Extension		
Prime	Gluteus maximus	
	Hamstrings	
Accessory	Ischial head of	L4, 5, S1, 2
	adductor magnus	
Abduction		
Prime	Gluteus medius	
Accessory	Gluteus minimus	L4, 5, S1
Adduction		
Prime	Adductor magnus	
	Adductor longus	
	Adductor brevis	L3, 4, 5, S1
	Pectineus	
	Gracilis	
External rotation		
Prime	Gluteus maximus	
	Quadratus femoris	
	Piriformis	L4, 5, S1
Accessory	Sartorius	
	Gracilis	
Internal rotation		
Prime	Gluteus minimus	
Accessory	Gluteus medius	
	Adductor longus	
	Adductor brevis	L4, 5, S1
	Adductor magnus	
	Pectineus	
	Iliacus	
	Psoas	

groin, inner thigh, trochanteric area, buttock, anterior thigh and knee (Figs 8.4–8.6). The reason why patients may present with knee pain is that both the hip and the knee receive a nerve supply from the obturator nerve and the femoral nerve. Pain from the joint therefore needs to be differentiated from referred pain from lumbar spinal disease and meralgia paraesthetica, and from that due to sacroiliitis, trochanteric bursitis, ischial bursitis and adductor tendinitis (Fig. 8.5).

In diseases of the articular surface, pain is often aggravated by weight-bearing. Pain due to joint inflammation is accompanied by prolonged stiffness and is often relieved by holding the leg in slight flexion if the joint capsule is distended. Pain resulting from joint infection or bone disease such as osteoid osteoma is often worse at night. The pain of bursitis is usually more localised. Trochanteric bursitis often causes deep aching over the lateral, upper thigh which is

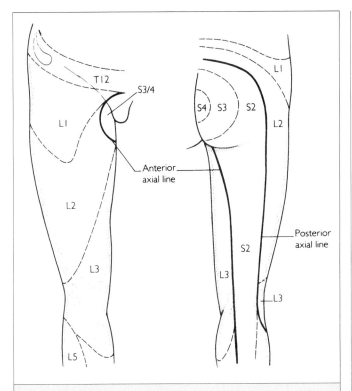

Fig. 8.3 Dermatomes of the lower extremity.

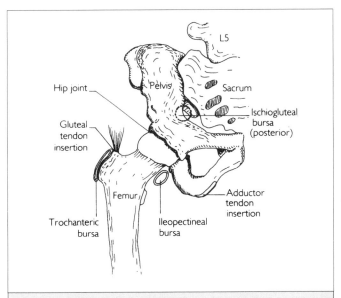

Fig. 8.4 Anatomical sites of pain arising from the hip joint.

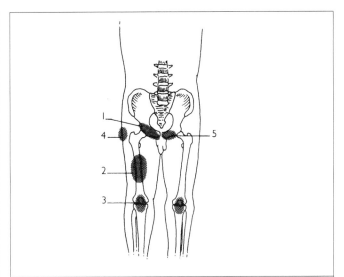

Fig. 8.5 *Hip disease* may cause diffuse pain and tenderness in the groin (1), and pain may radiate to the thigh (2) or knee (3); *trochanteric bursitis* causes pain and tenderness (4), and *gluteal tendinitis* may cause pain in the same area on resisted abduction; *adductor tendinitis* causes pain in the groin on resisted adduction (5); *meralgia paraesthetica* causes pain and dysaesthesia in a patch on the front of the thigh (2).

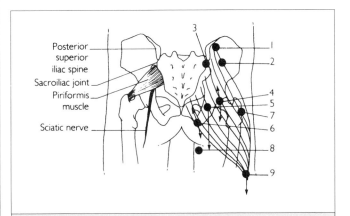

Fig. 8.6 Posterior view of hip; note the gluteus maximus attaching to the iliotibial tract: (1) gluteus medius bursa; (2) gluteus medius and maximus trigger point; (3) sacroiliac joint; (4) hip joint; (5) sciatic nerve; (6) ischiogluteal bursa; (7) trochanteric bursa; (8) adductor tendons; (9) iliotibial tract.

EXAMINATION

Inspection

The patient is undressed to underpants and examined walking, standing and lying. Easily identifiable bony landmarks of the pelvis and femur (Fig. 8.7) are the crest of the ilium, which terminates anteriorly at the anterior superior spine and posteriorly at the posterior superior spine, the ischial tuberosity and the greater trochanter. Anteriorly, the hip joint is beneath a point 3 cm below the midpoint of the

intensified by walking; it is often bad at night, being aggravated by lying on the affected side. Ischiogluteal bursitis ('Weaver's bottom') causes pain over the ischial tuberosity which is worse when sitting.

Fig. 8.7 Anatomical landmarks of the pelvis and femur.

inguinal ligament and 3 cm lateral to the palpable femoral artery.

Walking into the clinic the patient may give away the presence of hip disease. An antalgic gait indicates a painful hip. During the phase of gait when weight-bearing is on the affected side, the body leans over to the affected side to avoid painful contraction of the hip abductors. A Trendelenburg gait, on the other hand, indicates weakness of the abductor muscles, which is a frequent occurrence in any chronic hip disease. Here the pelvis on the opposite side drops and the body leans away from the affected side when weight-bearing is on the diseased hip. A waddling gait due to bilateral chronic hip disease and abductor muscle weakness is very typical of bilateral congenital hip displacement.

With the patient standing it is helpful to have him or her point to the site of pain. From the front, a pelvic tilt can be detected from the level of the anterior iliac spines (Fig. 8.8). This is due to adduction or abduction deformity resulting from hip disease, a short leg or primary scoliosis. External rotation, which is common in severe osteoarthritis or femoral neck fracture, may be apparent. From the side (Fig. 8.8(b)) an exaggerated lumbar lordosis may be an indication

(a) (b) (c)

Fig. 8.8 Inspection of the patient standing will detect pelvic tilt (a), exaggerated lumbar lordosis (b) and elevation of the iliac crest and gluteal fold (c).

of a fixed flexion deformity of one or both hips. From behind (Fig. 8.8(c)), elevation of the iliac crest and the gluteal fold on one side may indicate hip deformity. With fixed adduction, the diseased side is elevated and the patient may be unable to stand with the foot of the involved leg flat on the floor. With an abduction deformity the situation is reversed. Muscle wasting may be apparent, as the result of disuse in hip disease or due to primary neurological or muscle involvement.

The *Trendelenburg test* (Fig. 8.9) detects weakness of the gluteus medius hip abductors. This can be due to a variety of chronic hip diseases or to primary neurological or muscle disorders. The patient is asked to stand on the affected hip. Normally, the centre of gravity is brought over the weight-bearing foot and the abductor muscles hold the pelvis level or even with the non-supporting side slightly elevated. A positive test is indicated by dropping of the non-weight-bearing side.

When the patient is lying supine with the pelvis as level as possible, leg-length discrepancy will be obvious. Measuring each leg from the anterior iliac spine to the medial malleolus will indicate true leg shortening. A difference of less than 1 cm is quite commonly encountered and does not produce a functional problem. With a fixed adduction deformity, the affected leg may cross the normal one. Rotational deformities may be obvious and an inflamed, painful hip tends to be held in slight flexion, abduction and external rotation.

The hip joint is deep-seated and joint swelling is not usually apparent. Occasionally, swelling of the iliopectineal bursa can be seen in the medial part of the groin.

Palpation

Use the inguinal ligament (anterior superior iliac spine to pubis) and femoral artery as landmarks. Below the middle third of the inguinal ligament and just lateral to the femoral artery pulse, the anterior part of the hip joint can be palpated where a small part of the head lies outside the acetabulum. Overlying this is the iliopectineal bursa. Tenderness at this site (Fig. 8.10) may be due to joint inflammation or bursitis. Swelling of the iliopectineal bursa may be felt and is usually tender. This may be due to a localised bursitis or

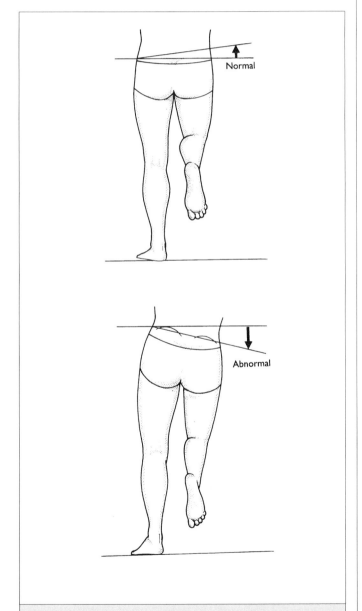

Fig. 8.9 The Trendelenburg test. When the gluteus medius is weak the pelvis drops on the non-weight-bearing side when the patient stands on the affected hip (lower).

Fig. 8.10 Palpate the hip joint and associated iliopectineal bursa by placing the fingers over the head of the femur below the inguinal ligament, lateral to the femoral artery.

may represent a synovial cyst through communication with an underlying inflamed hip joint. Swelling of the bursa must be distinguished from other swellings in this region, particularly from a femoral hernia that lies medial to the femoral artery.

Localised tenderness approximately 10 cm below the anterior superior iliac crest, at the point where the lateral cutaneous nerve of the thigh penetrates the deep fascia, is typical of meralgia paraesthetica. This is an entrapment neuropathy of this nerve.

By flexing and abducting the hip (Fig. 8.11), tenderness due to adductor tendinitis can be detected. Tenderness around the symphysis pubis and inferior pubic ramus occurs in spondylarthropathies as a result of enthesitis.

Turn the patient on his or her side to palpate the greater trochanter. Bursitis causes tenderness over the lateral aspect of the greater trochanter and occasionally there is swelling. Tenderness of the tendon insertions occurs on the posterolateral aspect of the greater trochanter. To palpate the ischial tuberosity, flex the hip and knee (Fig. 8.12). Tenderness may indicate bursitis, and rheumatoid nodules may be felt at this site. The sciatic nerve can be palpated midway between the greater trochanter and the ischial tuberosity and is tender in conditions putting pressure on it, such as intervertebral disc disease.

With the leg extended, percussion of the heel of the foot with the examiner's hand can produce pain in the hip in early cases of hip disease (the 'anvil' test).

Fig. 8.12 Palpation of the ischial tuberosity.

Range of movements

Except for testing extension, movements of the hip are best determined with the patient lying supine. The normal range of movements varies from person to person.

Thomas' test indicates a fixed flexion deformity of the hip (Fig. 8.13). Flex the good hip fully, observing with the other hand that the lumbar spine is flattened. Lifting of the thigh on the affected side with flexion of the knee indicates a positive test. A potential trap for the inexperienced clinician is the patient with a painful knee that is held in flexion. Although attempts to straighten the knee at the couch cause pain the knee otherwise appears normal. The problem here is a diseased hip with a fixed flexion deformity and pain

Fig. 8.11 Palpation of the origin of the adductor longus.

Fig. 8.13 Thomas' test.

referred to the knee. This becomes apparent when the examiner is able to extend the knee while flexing the hip; if the patient is seated (hip flexed) the knee can also be extended fully.

The range of flexion (approximately 120°) is tested with the knees flexed. Flexion of the hip with the knee extended is limited by tension in the hamstrings and varies considerably from person to person, from over 90° to less than 75°.

Abduction is frequently lost in hip disease. Test this with the legs extended by stabilising the pelvis with a hand on the opposite anterior iliac crest (Fig. 8.14) and grasping the ankle with the other hand. The hip is abducted until the pelvis tilts (approximately 45°). Additionally, the examiner can stand at the end of the couch to grasp both ankles and simultaneously abduct both hips: one can better appreciate differences between the two hips and measure the intermalleolar distance for future comparison. Adduction is assessed by crossing one leg over the other; normally, approximately 30° is possible before the pelvis tilts.

Loss of internal rotation is one of the earliest and most reliable signs of hip disease. Test this by flexing the hip and knee to 90° and rotate the foot laterally (Fig. 8.15). Normally there is about 45° of internal rotation but this is reduced with ageing; therefore a difference between the two sides is important. External rotation (approximately 45°, Fig. 8.16) is tested by rotating the foot medially. A rough idea of internal and external rotation and a comparison between the two sides can be achieved with the legs extended (Fig. 8.17), rolling each leg first one way then the other.

Extension of the hip is checked with the patient lying prone. The examiner partially immobilises the pelvis and lumbar spine by applying downward pressure with one hand while extending the hip with the other hand placed on the anterior aspect of the thigh.

Fig. 8.15 Testing internal rotation at 90° flexion. Measure the range of internal rotation by comparing the position of the leg and the midline. The normal range is 45°. Compare the two sides. Loss of internal rotation is common in most hip pathology.

Fig. 8.16 Testing external rotation at 90° flexion. The position of the hip is the same as for testing internal rotation but in this case the foot is moved medially.

Fig. 8.14 Abduction of the hip.

Pain on resisted movements in association with localised pain and tenderness indicate a tendinitis. For example, pain on resisted adduction and resisted abduction is typical of adductor tendinitis and gluteal tendinitis, respectively.

The *Ober test* demonstrates contraction of the iliotibial band. The patient lies on his or her side and the lower hip is flexed to eliminate lordosis of the lumbar spine. The knee of the upper leg is flexed to 90° and the thigh is abducted and extended. In a positive test, when the examiner's

Fig. 8.17 Testing rotation of the hip with the leg extended. Roll each leg medially and laterally and compare the sides.

Fig. 8.18 Assessing the strength of the lateral rotators of the hip.

Fig. 8.19 Testing the abductors of the hip.

Fig. 8.20 Testing the adductors of the hip.

supporting hand is removed, the hip remains abducted rather than dropping back to the couch and the iliotibial band is often palpated as a rigid band in the subcutaneous tissues below the iliac crest.

Muscle testing

Flexors of the hip are best tested with the patient sitting with his or her legs hanging over the couch. The hip is then actively flexed against graded resistance. The internal and external rotators are then tested with one of the examiner's hands applying counter-pressure to the thigh and the other hand applying graded resistance above the ankle against the movement being tested (Fig. 8.18).

Abductors and abductors are tested with the patient on one side with legs extended. For the abductors (Fig. 8.19), the lower leg is slightly flexed to maintain balance, the pelvis is stabilised with one hand, the upper leg is extended slightly and the patient abducts the leg against resistance provided by the examiner's other hand.

To test the adductors (Fig. 8.20), the upper leg is supported in approximately 30° of abduction, and adduction of the lower leg is resisted by the examiner with the other hand above the knee.

Testing the extensors is performed with the patient prone and the legs extended. With one hand on the sacrum to hold the pelvis down, the examiner resists extension of the hip with the other hand above the knee.

LOCAL ASPIRATION AND INJECTION

Hip joint

Aspiration of the hip joint requires more skill than other sites because the joint is deep to the skin surface so that one is unable to feel the articulation between the bones and often unable to confirm that the needle is in the joint space. The procedure is easier if fluoroscopy is available.

Figure 8.21 shows the anterior approach. The needle is inserted two fingers width lateral to the femoral artery, just below the inguinal ligament.

Bursitis

Trochanteric bursitis

With the affected side uppermost and flexed, and the lower leg extended on the couch, identify the tender site over the trochanteric prominence. The needle is inserted perpendicular to the skin until the trochanter is reached and then with-drawn slightly. The injection site can be very deep, especially in patients with obese thighs, and a 21-gauge needle is often required.

Ischiogluteal bursitis

With the patient lying on his or her side, facing away from the examiner, locate the site of greatest tenderness, and inject into this.

Meralgia paraesthetica (Fig. 8.22)

Locate the tender spot where the lateral cutaneous nerve of the thigh penetrates the fascia of the upper thigh approximately 10 cm below the anterior superior iliac spine. This site is then infiltrated. (Note: this is not the only site where compression may occur.)

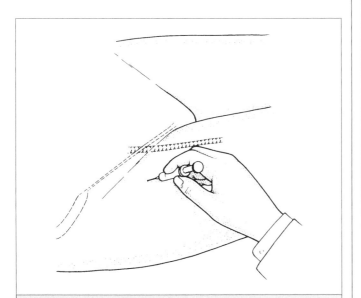

Fig. 8.21 Aspiration of the hip joint. Marks on the skin overlie the anterior superior spine, the greater trochanter, the femoral artery and the inguinal ligament. The needle is inserted two fingers width lateral to the femoral artery, just below the inguinal ligament.

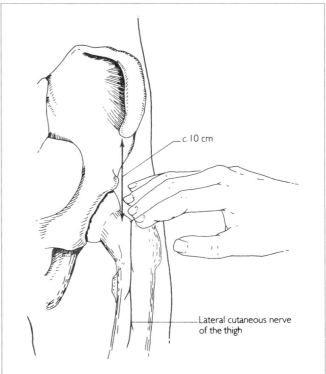

c. 10 cm

Lateral cutaneous nerve of the thigh

Fig. 8.22 Localising the site of injection in meralgia paraesthetica.

9

The knee

The knee is the largest and most complicated joint in the body and is a modified hinge joint with two tibiofemoral components and one patellofemoral. In some lower mammals, three distinct synovial cavities are found.

The knee is not constrained by the shape of its bones; it depends for stability on internal (cruciates and menisci) and external soft tissues (capsule and capsular ligaments) and muscle function/coordination. Nevertheless, the knee remains relatively unstable and is the joint most susceptible to injury, osteochondritis dissecans, loose bodies and synovial chondromatosis. The peripheral joint involvement of the seronegative spondarthritides typically includes the knee and symmetrical knee joint synovitis in rheumatoid arthritis is common.

It is the easiest joint to aspirate and a common target site for most arthropathies. It is therefore a frequent site for diagnostic aspiration.

DEVELOPMENT

Prenatal development

The development of the knee has been studied more than that of any other joint. By approximately 8 weeks it resembles that of the adult in form, the patella being cartilaginous by 10 weeks. The cruciate ligaments and menisci develop *in situ* and are not therefore secondary capsular structures. The characteristic feature of synovial tissue in the fetus is a vascularised loose connective tissue, covered by synovial cells of varied arrangements. A fibrous capsule is present only in the posterior part of the joint, and its appearance is so variable that it does not appear a necessary prelude to the formation of intra-articular structures.

Developmental abnormalities

The knee is commonly the site of abnormality in the disorders of epiphyseal growth. Where such a disorder is suspected it is essential to assess the whole skeletal system, to compare the findings with normal clinical and radiological charts and then refer to one of the specialist texts (e.g. *Atlas of Skeletal Dysplasias*). *Genu varum* or *valgum* (see Fig. 9.5) may be found according to the main site of epiphyseal maldevelopment. Where major laxity is a feature, recurvatum is likely.

Minor genu varum is common in normal children before the age of 3 years, and genu valgum may continue until 7 years. Severe genu valgum is seen in *Morquio's* syndrome due to failure of ossification of the lateral side of the upper tibial epiphyses. *Hypochondroplasia* (prevalence 3–4 per million), when severe, is indistinguishable from *achondroplasia*, but the only lower limb finding in the mild form may be genu varum (8% of cases).

Pseudoachondroplasia (prevalence 4 per million), unlike achondroplasia, causes marked epiphyseal and metaphyseal involvement, leading to premature osteoarthritis.

In *Marfan's syndrome* there is joint laxity and knee recurvatum, in addition to the long bone excess.

FUNCTIONAL ANATOMY

The knee is a modified hinge joint that also shows gliding and rotation of the articular surfaces on each other. The femoral condyles are *convex*, accentuated posteriorly. The tibial condyles are hollowed centrally but flattened peripherally so that concavity is produced by the overlying semilunar cartilages (*menisci*). Stability is therefore provided by the internal (*cruciate ligaments* and *menisci*) and external (*capsule* and *capsular ligaments*) soft tissues, including coordinated muscle function.

Menisci

The menisci (Fig. 9.1) or semilunar cartilages, are crescent-shaped portions of fibrocartilage, producing concavity by their situation on the upper articular surface of the tibia. Since they are wedge-shaped in cross-section, they match the adjacent articular surfaces of the femur and tibia.

Meniscal function

The menisci have a mild stabilising effect, exert some restriction on excessive lateral movement and facilitate the 'screw-home' movement. They act as 'thrust pads' aiding lubrication. They also play an important role in load-bearing, transmitting up to 70% of weight in extension through the lateral side and 50% medially.

Fibrous capsule

There is no defined complete capsule, but rather a thick ligamentous sheath comprising mainly tendons or expansions from them.

Anterior

- Fused tendons of the rectus femoris and vasti insert into the upper patella, with superficial fibres continuing over the anterior patella into the ligamentum patellae.

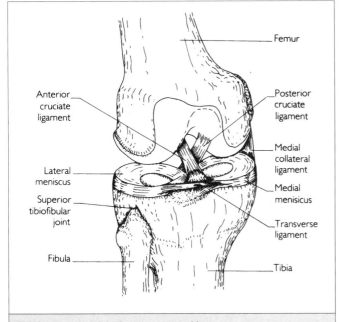

Fig. 9.1 Interior of the knee: menisci and ligaments.

Labels: Femur; Anterior cruciate ligament; Posterior cruciate ligament; Medial collateral ligament; Lateral meniscus; Medial meniscus; Superior tibiofibular joint; Transverse ligament; Fibula; Tibia.

- Thinner bands from the sides of the patella attach to the anterior border of each tibial condyle (*medial and lateral patellar retinacula*).
- Strong expansions of fascia lata lie more superficially (*iliotibial tract*), descending over the anterolateral knee to the lateral tibial condyle, with a band to the lateral upper patella (*superior patellar retinaculum*).

Note: Unlike other hinge joints the 'capsule' is continuous with the muscle above, so its tension can be fully modified in all positions.

Posterior

- True capsular fibres attach to the femur above the condyles and to the intercondylar line, vertically down to the upper tibia.
- Centrally strengthened by the *oblique popliteal ligament*.
- Inferolaterally by the *arcuate popliteal ligament*.

Medial

- The true capsular fibres form the *superficial collateral ligament*, which is broad and flat attaching to the medial epicondyle of the femur, passing down and slightly forwards to the medial tibia (superficial to below tibial tubercle, deep also to medial meniscus).
- Expansions of the *semimembranosus tendon* add considerable strength to the medial and posterior capsule.

Lateral

- The *fibular collateral ligament* is round and cord-like, separated from the lateral capsule and enclosed by an expansion of fascia lata. It splits the tendon of biceps femoris.
- The popliteus tendon lies between the lateral meniscus and capsule.

Note: the collateral ligaments are most tightly stretched in extension and their lines of attachment prevent rotation of the tibia laterally or of the femur medially in extension. Rotation is easily demonstrated in the flexed knee.

Intra-articular ligaments

These are called *cruciates* as they cross each other within the joint.

Anterior cruciate (ACL)

This extends obliquely up and back from the anterior intercondylar area of the tibia to the medial aspect of the lateral femoral condyle. Thus it prevents posterior displacement of the femur on the tibia.

Posterior cruciate (PCL)

This is less oblique, shorter and stronger. It passes up and forwards from the posterior intercondylar area of the tibia medial to the ACL, and attaches to the lateral side of the medial femoral condyle. It prevents anterior displacement of the femur on the tibia.

These ligaments are more taut in extension and tend to rotate the tibia laterally. They tighten when the tibia is rotated medially and slacken when rotated laterally as the ligaments uncross.

Extensor mechanism (Fig.9. 2)

Extension is by the quadriceps femoris, which is one of the most powerful muscles in the body. It is formed by the rectus femoris and three vasti (medialis, intermedius and lateralis), and extends the knee and flexes the hip.

Any injury to the knee joint produces inhibition of this muscle, which rapidly loses bulk, tone and control, especially seen in the vastus medialis obliquus (VMO). The VMO is the most important component and contributes to medial stability of the patella and the 'screw home' movement of the femur on the tibia in the last 10° of extension.

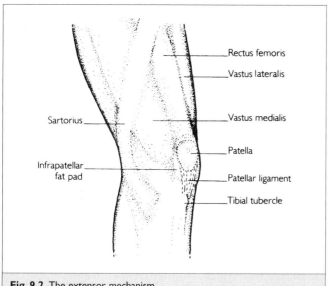

Fig. 9.2 The extensor mechanism.

The *patellar ligament* is an extension of the quadriceps (patellar) tendon from the inferior patellar pole to its insertion into the tibial tubercle. The infrapatellar fat pad can be seen on either side of the ligament, as it lies behind the ligament, separating it from the synovial membrane.

Knee flexion is performed by the hamstrings (biceps femoris, semimembranosus and semitendinosus) and gastrocnemii.

- *The biceps femoris* by its insertion to fibular head, fibular collateral ligament, iliotibial tract and upper tibia and deep fascia of the calf, flexes the knee and gives lateral dynamic support.
- *The semimembranosus*, by its insertion to posterior and medial tibial condyle and post capsule, flexes and gives posterior and medial stability. Its tendon extends across the posterior aspect from the medial tibial condyle upwards to the lateral femoral condyle as the *posterior oblique ligament*.
- *The semitendinosus* joins the sartorius to insert into the upper and medial tibial shaft and *gracilis* (pes anserinus).

Rotation

Rotation is not possible in the fully extended stable knee; but as the knee flexes, medial rotation is performed by the sartorius, gracilis, semimembranosus and semitendinosus. Lateral rotation is carried out by the biceps femoris and tensor fasciae latae.

Rotatory stability

Rotatory stability is provided by the popliteus, which is a medial rotator of the tibia on the femur and protects the posterolateral portion of the lateral meniscus, because the tendon attaches to the lateral meniscus and pulls it back during knee flexion and medial rotation.

Medial stability

Medial stability (Fig. 9.3) is achieved by the function of the medial collateral ligament, which is a primary static stabiliser, and the semimembranosus muscle, which is a dynamic stabiliser. The medial tibial collateral ligament is phylogenetically a continuation of the insertion of the adductor magnus. It comprises a superficial portion, a deep portion (from the joint capsule and attaching to the periph-

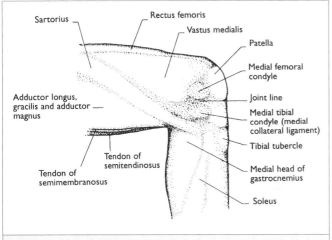

Fig. 9.3 Surface anatomy of the medial aspect of the knee. (Structures providing medial stability highlighted.)

eral medial meniscus) and an oblique portion which is fan-shaped from the medial femoral condyle to the posterior aspect of the medial tibial condyle and peripheral medial meniscus. The oblique portion remains tight in flexion, when the posterior capsule is very lax.

Lateral stability

Lateral stability (Fig. 9.4) is achieved by the function of the lateral (fibular) collateral ligament as a static stabiliser and the biceps femoris muscle as a dynamic stabiliser. The lateral

collateral ligament is phylogenetically the origin of the peroneus longus, and it extends from the lateral epicondyle of the femur down to the head of the fibula. It splits the tendon of the biceps femoris and is separated from the lateral meniscus by the tendon of popliteus.

Innervation

The knee joint is supplied by several branches of the femoral nerve, the common peroneal and tibial (sciatic) nerves and a filament from the obturator nerve. The latter explains the common referral, particularly in children, of the pain of hip joint disease to the knee, typically medially.

Vascular supply

There are branches from the popliteal, anterior tibial and a descending branch from the lateral circumflex femoral branch of the arteria profunda femoris.

PAIN PATTERNS IN THE KNEE

It is necessary to define whether symptoms are spontaneous or post-traumatic. The features of inflammatory or degenerative joint disease have been outlined in Chapter 1.

Osteoarthritis

Pain is usually first noticed on exercise, but can initially be 'walked off'. The patient may complain that the knee creaks and grates, with episodes of swelling, particularly after unusual activity in a flexed position (e.g. squatting or kneeling). The swelling and a variable degree of inflammatory response in the synovium produces a stiff, tight feeling (*inactivity stiffness*), felt particularly at the back of the knee. Sudden increase in stress may precipitate acute pain. Cartilage or osteophytic fragments which separate into the joint may cause loose body *locking*. Flexion deformity occurs due to protective hamstring spasm, but will in time become a fixed flexion deformity.

In the later stages, pain becomes more severe and near constant, with progressive genu varum. The patient becomes unable to squat or kneel and has difficulty climbing stairs.

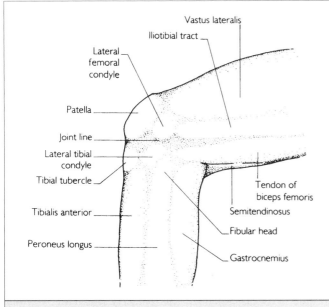

Fig. 9.4 Surface anatomy of the lateral aspect of the knee.

Synovitis

The patient complains of pain and stiffness with marked morning symptoms. Tightness at the back of the knee may be very limiting, particularly if there is a tense popliteal cyst. If the effusion is very tense, flexion is often very restricted and extension difficult due to hamstring tightness. Flexion contracture will develop if the effects are not reduced by reduction of synovitis and splintage.

HISTORY OF INJURY

It is important to define the history of the plane and forces of injury.

Acute injury

A team doctor, coach or physiotherapist may be able to describe the observed forces of injury. It is vital to examine the injured knee immediately, before protective muscle spasm makes this impossible. *Immediate swelling* indicates a haemarthrosis and demands urgent investigation to determine whether it is due to cruciate ligament tear, osteochondral injury or other pathology.

Chronic injury

The history of the type of injury may be the main pointer to the likely damage, as physical signs are often of limited value. The patient should be asked to describe or demonstrate the pattern of injury. Where no defined injury is recalled, the loading, type of training and surfaces used should be defined.

An alternative pathology must be considered if the symptoms and signs do not fit with the stresses involved.

Anterior knee pain

Pain is felt behind the knee cap, particularly after sitting with the knee flexed for some time (cinema sign), and is relieved by movement but aggravated by heavy exercise, especially loaded in flexion. There is pain particularly when descending stairs. This is because of increased stress on this compartment when maintaining knee flexion or particularly when weight-bearing on a flexed knee.

In the examination:

- the findings are often minimal,
- there may be tenderness of the medial patella undersurface,
- fluid and crepitus may be present in chondromalacia patellae if severe,
- VMO wasting.

'Giving way' due to patellar subluxation

The patella functions in a state of dynamic equilibrium between lateral forces (vastus lateralis, bony contour and position of tibial tubercle and genu valgum) and medial forces (patella alta, ligamentous laxity and vastus medialis) (see patella Q-angle, Fig. 8.12).

In *mild* patellar subluxation, the patella slips momentarily over the condyle. The patient describes the history of 'giving way' and may develop mild synovitis or effusion after each episode, if infrequent. Frequent displacement is, on the other hand, often pain-free.

The patellar apprehension test: the examiner pushes the patella laterally with the knee in extension; as the knee is flexed actively, the patient resists further flexion because of fear of painful dislocation. A positive test is strong evidence of recurrent dislocation in patients presenting with a history of recurrent 'giving way' of the knee. However, apprehension may also be seen in individuals complaining of patellofemoral pain without a history of 'giving way'.

In *major* subluxation with severe pain, reduction under general anaesthesia is usually necessary when the episode is the first and caused by direct injury. Arthroscopy should be performed to exclude injury to the patella surface, since later symptoms resulting from a detached osteochondral fragment may develop.

Vastus medialis obliquus wasting is often a prominent finding in patients with patellar abnormalities.

Medial meniscal tear

Acute: there is usually a history of an outward twist of foot/ankle or an inward twist of femur on fixed foot with the knee in flexion. Immediate anteromedial pain is often sufficient to make the individual collapse. There may have been a feeling of a tearing sensation inside the joint. On attempting to stand, the knee usually cannot be straightened *if* there is displacement of the meniscal segment. Swelling develops a few hours later (*unless* there is a peripheral tear in the vascular portion or an associated cruciate tear, when immediate swelling, due to haemarthrosis, occurs). With a mild tear the symptoms tend to improve over the following week but chronic symptoms may be noted, particularly if squatting or turning.

Chronic: the patient can usually walk and carry out normal activities, but any twisting movement gives pain or *giving way of the knee*. Locking episodes and recurrent small effusions may also be noticed, but persistent effusion is relatively uncommon. Quadriceps wasting is common.

Lateral meniscal tear

The history is usually similar except that the pain is often felt posteriorly, locking is less frequent and the injury sometimes remains asymptomatic. A posterior tear produces pain at the end of knee flexion, which may be limited, and a click may be felt.

Locked knee

Locking refers to the inability to fully extend the knee (*blocked knee*) due to a meniscal tear, or to hyperextend it if it normally does. *Fixed flexion deformity* is the clinical sign (Fig. 9.5) and the affected knee should be compared with the normal one. Extension to neutral (0°) may still indicate a blocked knee if the opposite knee hyperextends (i.e. if the affected knee previously hyperextended). Fixed flexion deformity of the knee not associated with acute injury may be secondary to hip flexion deformity or to hamstring contraction. *Locking* due to a *loose body*, occurs suddenly in mid-movement and prevents extension or flexion. Sudden intense pain may cause the patient to fall. Typically, the site of pain is variable. Recurrent episodes may lead to chronic synovitis and effusion.

EXAMINATION

As with all lower limb joints, assessment should begin with observation of standing posture, gait and leg length. Observe the alignment between the lower leg (tibia) and upper leg (femur).

Genu varum (Fig. 9.5)

Genu varum refers to lateral curvature of the leg involving tibia or tibia and femur:

- *Tibia: physiological tibial bowing* refers to minor bowing, which is common before the age of 3 years; it corrects with further growth. *Pathological tibial bowing* results from rickets, typically in the distal third, trauma or infection.
- *Tibia/femur*: congenital genu varum occurs because of abnormalities in epiphyseal growth. In osteoarthritis genu varum develops when there is loss of the medial compartment cartilage and ligament laxity.

Genu valgum (Fig. 9.5)

- *Physiological* genu valgum resolves by the age of 7 years.
- *Unilateral* genu valgum may be due to trauma, infections or congenital causes affecting epiphyseal growth.
- *Bilateral (or unilateral)* genu valgum is usually a result of inflammatory joint disease, for example rheumatoid arthritis.

Genu recurvatum

This is hyperextension of the knee beyond 10° (Fig. 9.5) and may be part of a generalised hypermobility syndrome or have localised causes, including underdevelopment of the femoral condyles or relaxation of the posterior capsular structures and weakness in the calf and hamstring muscles.

Muscle wasting

Observe the quadriceps muscle bulk, the vastus medialis obliquas; particularly since it wastes rapidly in any painful knee condition. Exclude evidence of denervation, root irritation (positive femoral stretch test) or primary muscle disease (myopathy/myositis). Observe for fasciculation as a sign of denervation, particularly in diabetic amyotrophy. Compare

Fig. 9.5 Genu varum (a), valgum (b), recurvatum (c) and fixed flexion (d).

muscle strength in quadriceps with hamstrings, as *imbalance* may be the cause of persistent problems, particularly in sportsmen.

A tape-measure record of muscle wasting can be made by a circumferential measure at a point (6–10 cm) measured and marked above the superior patellar pole on both sides (Fig. 9.6). Reproducibility is rather poor, but serial measurements may have some value in monitoring recovery of muscle bulk. *Maximum* calf circumference is more reproducible, but is of more value in defining venous calf distension or popliteal cyst leakage.

Swelling

Define whether there is *generalised* (e.g. effusion or soft tissue) or *localised* (e.g. meniscal or bursal) swelling.

Effusion

This fills in the parapatellar gutters and suprapatellar pouch, but also examine for popliteal swelling. A small effusion is best defined by the *bulge test*. Fluid is stroked by the palm of the (right) hand from the medial joint line (start at tibial condyle) upwards into the suprapatellar pouch (Fig. 9.7). The (left) hand is immediately placed across the upper medial line with the thumb resting on the patella, thus controlling the fluid in the pouch and patellar movement. The fluid is then stroked down from the suprapatellar pouch by the dorsum of the right hand running down the lateral joint line.

A bulge of fluid at the medial patellar gutter confirms a small effusion (Fig. 9.7(d)). This must be defined from movement of the patella or soft tissues, but this should be controlled by the thumb resting on the patella.

A large effusion can be defined by cross-fluctuance (Fig. 9.8) or the patellar tap test, provided that the effusion has not become very tense.

The patellar tap (Fig. 9.9): the left hand controls the effusion by pressure over the suprapatellar pouch, while the right hand (index and middle fingers) taps the patella against the underlying femur by a sharp downward pressure with the knee in extension.

Synovitis can be crudely assessed by palpating the thickness of tissue in the suprapatellar pouch below the main quadriceps bulk, or by palpating swelling at the anterior joint line, which immediately reforms after pressure although this may be simulated by fat.

Localised swelling

The examiner should define

- anatomical site,
- communication with the knee joint,
- reducibility,
- consistency,
- tenderness,
- transillumination,
- and also exclude pulsation (also examine for bruit).

Meniscal cysts

Observe for swelling at the medial or lateral joint line (Figs 9.3 and 9.4). A cyst is usually quite tense and tender on local pressure. However, swelling may be intermittent, being more obvious after activity and settling with rest.

Bursae

The bursae of the knee are illustrated in Figure 9.10.

Prepatellar: this is present in about 90% of people and is subcutaneous, covering the lower half of the patella and upper half of the patellar ligament. In *bursitis due to pressure/friction* effects (housemaid's or carpetlayer's knee), pain may be absent, tenderness mild and the swelling cool. In chronic lesions the bursa may be rather indurated and gritty. In *acute bursitis*, due to crystal synovitis or sepsis, warmth,

Fig. 9.6 Measurement of thigh circumference.

Fig. 9.7 The bulge test. (a), (b), (c) indicates order of actions. (d) Observe bulge under patella (small arrow)

Fig. 9.8 The 'balloon' sign demonstrated at the knee. With one hand pressing over the suprapatellar pouch, posterior pressure on the patella causes outward expansion of the other examining hand due to fluid confinement within the joint.

Fig. 9.9 The patellar tap test.

erythema and local tenderness are marked but full passive knee flexion may, however, still be possible, with discomfort at end-range, as the knee joint is not involved, being protected by dense ligamentous and fibrous structures. This is in contrast with the marked irritability and gross restriction of knee joint sepsis.

Fig. 9.10 Bursae of the knee.

Fig. 9.11 Popliteal (Baker's) cyst.

Deep infrapatellar: this small bursa lies between the upper part of the tibial tuberosity and the ligamentum patellae: it is separated from the knee joint synovium by a pad of fat. When it is inflamed, note the swelling on either side of the patellar ligament insertion to the tibial tubercle. There is pain and tenderness over the ligament, and full knee extension and flexion are not quite achieved.

Popliteus: this arises from the synovial membrane of the knee surrounding the popliteus tendon intra-articularly. When inflamed, it can be seen as a rounded swelling behind the lateral condyle of the femur, deep to biceps and the iliotibial band.

Bicipital: this is lower than the popliteus bursa, lying between the biceps tendon and the lateral ligament. It can be confused with a neuroma of the lateral popliteal nerve, although local pressure should produce paraesthesiae in the nerve distribution if a neuroma.

Anserine: this is under the pes anserinus and therefore liable to bursitis, e.g. in breast-stroke swimmers.

Semimembranosus: this lies between the head of gastrocnemius and semimembranosus, and becomes inflamed after excessive knee flexion (gamekeeper's knee). During extension the swelling is firm and tense, but in flexion it becomes soft. When it communicates with the posterior aspect of the knee joint it is usually termed a Baker's or popliteal cyst (Fig. 9.11), which is common with a large knee joint effusion as it develops at the weak point of the posterior knee joint.

Rupture of a popliteal cyst: presents with a typical history of sudden upper calf pain (the patient may describe the onset 'as if being kicked in the calf'), and reduction of knee swelling, followed by generalised calf swelling and often pitting oedema of the dorsum of the foot. The most important differential diagnosis is from deep vein thrombosis, and sometimes, owing to secondary venous obstruction, a deep vein thrombosis can develop after cyst rupture. A venogram is therefore the investigation of choice.

Iliotibial bursa cyst (see iliotibial band syndrome, p. 111.).

Local tenderness

Define the site—bony, soft-tissue attachment to bone (enthesis) of tendon or ligament, bursal (Fig. 9.10) or joint line. Define associated swelling, and pain on resisted muscle action. Prominence and tenderness at the tibial tubercle is seen particularly in apophysitis (Osgood–Schlatter's disease).

Patellar mechanism

Patellar position

The position of the patella is assessed by measurement of the Q-angle (Fig. 9.12), between the line drawn from the anterior superior iliac spine to the centre of the patella and the line of the patellar ligament to the tibial tubercle. The ratio of the patellar ligament length to patellar length should be *less than*

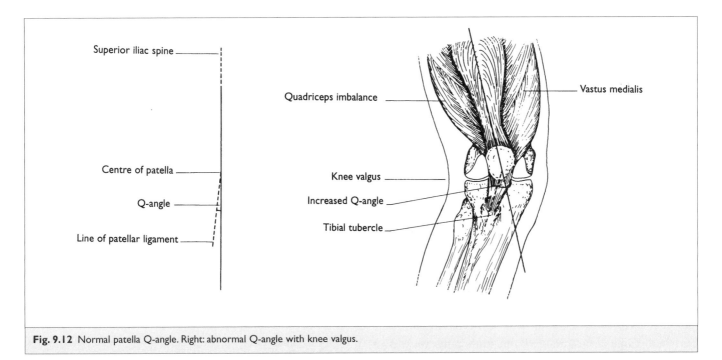

Fig. 9.12 Normal patella Q-angle. Right: abnormal Q-angle with knee valgus.

1.2:1.0. If greater this is referred to as patella alta and the patella is usually small.

The articular surface of the patella is divided into a large lateral section and smaller medial portion by a rounded vertical ridge. The cartilage cover of the most medial part of this area rests on the medial femoral condyle crescentic facet.

The patella tends to be displaced laterally during forced extension of the knee. This is counteracted by the buttress of the prominent lateral surface of the femur and by the retaining action of the lower fibres of vastus medialis which insert into the medial patellar border.

Abnormalities of patellar anatomy

Note any abnormalities, which include

- patella alta (high, and usually small, patella),
- patella baja (low patella),
- bipartite patella—a small gap may be palpable and this is usually bilateral,
- offset patella—due to an increased Q-angle. (Fig. 9.12)

A high patella and/or hypermobility predispose to patellar subluxation, which may follow a blow or commonly as the result of muscular action alone.

A patellar plica may be palpable, especially medially, and may be a cause of knee pain in athletes (see Fig. 9.22).

Range of movement and flexion deformity

Observe the position in which the knee is held. Flexion deformity or locked knee may be best detected by the prone-lying test (Fig. 9.13).

Quadriceps lag

Ask the patient to lift the lower limb off the couch with the knee extended. This will reveal any quadriceps lag, due to weakness. Then passively extend the knee and compare with the opposite knee. Define flexion deformity, and note that loss of hyperextension compared with the opposite side still implies a locked knee unless there is a cause for the unilateral excessive hyperextension. Then ask the patient to bend the knee as far as possible.

Fig. 9.13 Prone-lying test.

Flexion deformity

Define whether there is a bony or soft block to extension. The latter is a common sequel to chronic unopposed hamstring overaction with extensor weakness. Chronic hamstring tightness, particularly in sportsmen, may therefore produce flexion deformity with anterior knee pain. However, *spinal problems* may be the underlying reason for the hamstring tightness.

Always *exclude hip flexion deformity*, which results in secondary knee flexion deformity.

Locked knee

This is usually detected easily as already outlined or by using the prone-lying test (Fig. 9.13). It may be due to a meniscal tear. The site of pain on reaching the block to extension may localise the site of the tear. In a posterior horn tear of the lateral meniscus, there may be limited flexion and an audible or palpable 'clunk' on flexion. McMurray's test for meniscal injury (rotational stress while extending the knee from almost full flexion) is not recommended as it may be very painful (including patellofemoral stress) and risks locking the meniscal fragment.

A locked knee represents a surgical emergency because of the risk of further damage, including anterior cruciate rupture. Urgent arthroscopy is indicated.

Examination for stability

Test the integrity of the collateral ligaments with the knee flexed to about 20°. The examiner controls the patient's foot and ankle between the arms and chest wall and then applies a valgus or varus stress on the tibia. Separation of the tibia from the femur at the joint line should be checked for.

Medial collateral ligament

Valgus stretch is applied with the knee in flexion (Fig. 9.14) (if positive with the knee in extension, it denotes a posterior cruciate tear is also present). Minor symmetrical stretch is normal, with up to 5 mm separation. In medial ligament injury or lesions, the following patterns are found.

- *Mild (1st degree)*: there is a minimal tear with local tenderness and less than 5 mm separation (stable).
- *Moderate (2nd degree)*: there is a moderate tear with marked local tenderness and between 5 and 10 mm separation.

Fig. 9.14 The test of medial stability (arrow denotes direction of lateral stress).

- *Severe (3rd degree)*: there is more than 10 mm separation (unstable joint).

Lateral collateral ligament

Varus stretch is applied with knee in flexion (as medial). Injury to the lateral collateral ligament is much less common than injury to the medial since adduction stress in flexion is much less frequent in sport. If it occurs, the former is usually a complex injury, with lateral capsular ligament, biceps tendon, popliteus and occasionally iliotibial tract injury.

Anterior stability

Anterior cruciate tear is best defined by the Lachman's and pivot shift tests.

Lachman's test for anterior cruciate laxity (Fig. 9.15): with the knee flexed to 20–30°, the femur is grasped with the left hand and the tibia with the right. An attempt to pull the tibia forwards (on the femur) is then made.

Fig. 9.15 Lachman's test, shown in 20° flexion (arrow denotes direction of stress).

Pivot shift test (Fig. 9.16): the lower leg, with the foot internally rotated, is supported by the examiner while applying a valgus force, as the knee is flexed from *full* extension. A tear of the anterior cruciate, because it produces anterior subluxation of the tibia on the femur, causes a jump at about 30° when the tibia reduces as the knee is flexed, sliding backwards into its correct position on the femur.

Anterior drawer test (Fig. 9.17): the anterior drawer test is a less satisfactory test for anterior cruciate laxity but may have to be used by those finding the Lachman's test difficult to perform. With the knee in 90° of flexion, the examiner pulls forward with both hands on the upper posterior calf. Interpretation of the test is dependent on the position of the tibia in relation to femur. In the neutral position it tests the capsule and anterior cruciate. With the tibia in internal rota-

tion it tests the posterior cruciate (Fig. 9.16). A pure anterior drawer movement in neutral with the knee at 90° and relaxed hamstrings is termed the *anterior drawer sign*. When the tibia is internally rotated, the posterior cruciate is tight, so the anterior drawer movement cannot be achieved. Therefore a positive anterior drawer in internal rotation points to a torn posterior cruciate ligament. In summary, the following interpretations relate to a positive anterior test:

- in internal rotation—torn posterior cruciate;
- in neutral with equal tibial condyle movement—torn anterior cruciate with anteromedial/anterolateral laxity;
- in neutral with lateral tibial condyle movement—anterolateral (accentuated by the anterior cruciate) instability;
- in neutral with medial movement: anteromedial (accentuated by anterior cruciate), instability.

Posterior stability

The posterior drawer test is used when posterior cruciate tear is suspected. With the knee in 90° flexion, the alignment of the knee in relation to the femur is observed and compared with the opposite knee to see if there is posterior subluxation of the tibia. If there is subluxation, performing an anterior drawer test will correct this position to the normal (hence *posterior drawer sign*), thus distinguishing the signs from those of anterior cruciate rupture.

THE TIBIOFIBULAR JOINT

The tibia and fibula are connected at their upper and lower ends by joints—the *superior* and *inferior tibiofibular* joints —and their shafts are joined by the crural *interosseous membrane*.

The superior tibiofibular joint

This is a plane joint with flat oval articular surfaces (facets) between the lateral condyle of the tibia and the fibular head.

The *capsular ligament* attaches to the margins of the facets and is much thicker *anteriorly*. The synovial membrane of the joint may in some cases communicate with the knee joint through the popliteal bursa. The *anterior ligament* is two or three flat bands passing from the front of the fibular head obliquely upwards to the front of the lateral tibial condyle. The *posterior ligament* is a thick band from the back of the fibular head passing upwards obliquely to the posterior aspect of lateral tibial condyle.

Fig. 9.16 The pivot shift test. Note: the test begins in extension, the shift occurring as the knee is flexed. (Illustrates position when tibia reduces as the knee is flexed from full extension.) The arrow indicates the valgus force applied from extension on the internally rotated leg.

Fig. 9.17 The anterior drawer test (arrow denotes direction of pull).

The *anterior tibial vessels* pass between the tibia and fibula, through a gap in the upper interosseous membrane just below the fibular head.

The *lateral popliteal nerve* follows a line drawn from the apex of the popliteal fossa downwards and laterally along the medial side of the biceps tendon to the posterior head of the fibula—*it can be rolled against the bone at this site*. It lies between the biceps femoris tendon and lateral head of gastrocnemius, winding around the fibular neck deep to the peroneus longus and then divides into musculocutaneous and anterior tibial nerves.

Examination

Look for swelling by observing any difference between the two sides in the contour of the lateral aspects below the joint. This is best observed from *above* with the knees *flexed* to about 90°.

Palpate the joint line for tenderness and then assess laxity by pulling forward with three fingers pressing forward on the head and neck of the fibula. Note any sensory symptoms produced by these manoevres or by tapping the back of the fibular head (Tinel's test), indicating irritation of the lateral popliteal nerve.

LOCAL ASPIRATION AND INJECTION

Arthrocentesis of the knee joint

There are four major entry sites suitable for knee aspiration, medial retropatellar, lateral retropatellar, suprapatellar and anterior. Whatever the approach used, corticosteroids should only be injected into the joint if a clear diagnosis which justifies injection has been made. A strict aseptic technique is essential for any aspiration.

The knee is the easiest joint to enter and, since it is commonly affected by inflammatory joint disease and non-inflammatory effusions, it is the joint most frequently aspirated as a means of both diagnosis and treatment. The large capacity of the joint and the very large synovial surface area may result in huge effusions, but also a significant absorption of corticosteroid when injected into the joint, which may result in sufficient blood levels to produce a systemic 'steroid boost' effect. Aspiration to dryness may in itself give considerable pain relief and, where a large popliteal cyst has formed, removal of the fluid, allowing decompression of the cyst, may allow the knee to regain full extension.

Medial retropatellar approach

The medial approach is the easiest when there is a moderate or large effusion. This is performed with the patient lying supine on a firm couch with the lower limbs extended. It is essential to encourage the patient to relax, so that the quadriceps muscle is not tensed as this will clamp the patella down into the patellar groove, blocking needle introduction.

The site of entry medially (Fig. 9.18) is just below the midpoint of the patella. The needle is introduced in a line towards the suprapatellar pouch. It is important to aspirate back as the needle is progressed, as fluid may be found after/above only 1.5 cm of penetration. In this way, too deep introduction of the needle, with possible damage to the articular cartilage, will be avoided.

As the fluid is aspirated it can be 'milked down' by controlled pressure with one hand over the suprapatellar pouch.

Lateral retropatellar approach

The patient should lie flat and supine with the knee extended. The line of injection is at the point of the junction of the middle and upper thirds of the patella (Fig. 9.19). One hand can be placed on the inner aspect of the patella and used to slightly displace the patella laterally, which increases the gap between patella and femur laterally. The needle (21 gauge is usually sufficient) should be introduced at the junction point described above, upwards towards the suprapatellar pouch. As the needle is introduced, aspiration back should be performed and this will prevent pushing the needle too far (which usually means introduction into fatty tissue behind the suprapatellar pouch).

Fig. 9.18 Arthrocentesis of the left knee. Medial approach.

Fig. 9.19 Arthrocentesis of the left knee. Lateral approach.

Suprapatellar approach

If there is a very large effusion, expanding the suprapatellar bursa, the needle can be introduced into the suprapatellar pouch above and just lateral to the patella.

Anterior approach

An anterior approach, with the knee flexed to 90°, was favoured by some clinicians as it avoided the risk of needling articular cartilage, but it is now rarely used.

The needle is inserted just below the patellar pole and to the side of the patellar tendon. It is introduced parallel to the line of the tibial plateau, entering the intercondylar fossa between the medial and lateral condyles after 4–5 cm.

Corticosteroid injection

Where a clear diagnosis meriting corticosteroid injection has been made, a long-acting preparation, such as triamcinolone hexacetonide (20 mg) or methylprednisolone (80 mg) acetate, should be introduced. The patient should be advised to reduce walking and knee exercising for the immediate 24–48 hour period after injection, to reduce systemic absorption of the drug. Inpatient studies have shown that a 24 hour period of bed-rest improves the local benefit of injection.

Soft-tissue injection around the knee

Many painful soft-tissue conditions around the knee respond to local corticosteroid injection. However, a clear indication for injection must be confirmed and accurate anatomical localisation of the injection defined.

The most common conditions requiring injection and their localisation are described below. They are all best injected using a short-acting preparation (hydrocortisone acetate 25.0–37.5 mg) mixed with a small volume of lignocaine, provided that there is no history of previous allergic reaction.

Bursitis

It is essential that, if an infected bursa is suspected (usually prepatellar), the needle is *not* introduced into the knee joint itself, as this carries the risk of spreading infection into the joint. Even in a septic bursitis, fluid may not be obtained, but a small volume of local anaesthetic or sterile saline can be injected and then aspirated back to provide a specimen for culture.

The *prepatellar bursa* (Fig. 9.20) should be injected towards the centre of the maximum point of fluctuance, usually over or just below the lower portion of the patella, with the needle at an angle of about 30° to the skin.

The *deep infrapatellar bursa* should be approached from either the medial or lateral aspect and the needle directed deep to the patellar ligament, proximal to its insertion to the tibial tubercle. This may be enlarged due to Osgood–Schlatter's disease, previously with calcific debris behind the ligament irritating this and the bursa. Frequent recurrence despite injection should be treated surgically.

Attachment lesions in osteoarthritis of the knee

In osteoarthritis of the knee, pain is commonly localised to one of the collateral ligament attachments (usually the medial), and may be elicited by stress testing or by finding tenderness by pressing with one finger over the attachment (Fig. 9.21). Infiltration of the tender area with hydrocortisone is often very helpful, provided that there is no major instability.

In patellofemoral osteoarthritis, persistent and localised tender sites in the patellar retinaculum attachment to the patellar borders may respond to local injection, but the needle should not enter the joint. These tender sites must be localised accurately by displacing the patella with one hand and then palpating the patellar edge on the opposite side

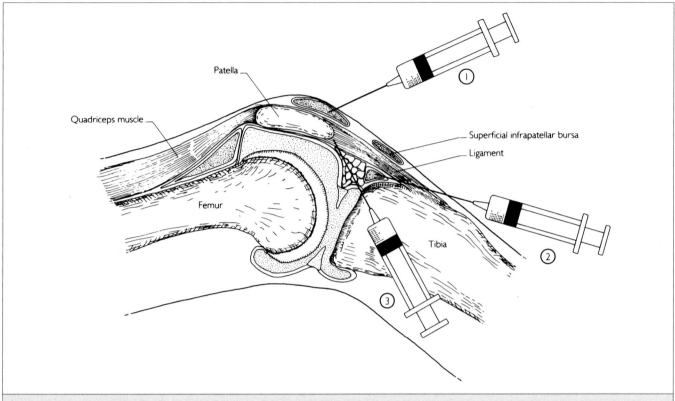

Fig. 9.20 Soft-tissue injection of the anterior structures of the knee. 1, Prepatellar bursa; 2, deep infrapatellar bursa; 3, patellar pole tendinitis.

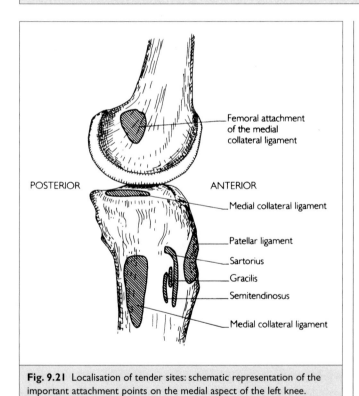

Fig. 9.21 Localisation of tender sites: schematic representation of the important attachment points on the medial aspect of the left knee.

medial aspect of the patella, should be excluded in the athlete. This has a synovial lining which may become inflamed due to overuse in sport, or in inflammatory joint disease. This usually responds to local hydrocortisone injection, but persistent plical tenderness and pain in an athlete may occasionally require arthroscopic excision.

Tendinitis

Chronic inflammation at the attachment of the patellar tendon (ligament) to the inferior patellar pole, and less commonly the superior patellar pole, usually responds well to local injection, provided that there is no deep-seated necrotic tendon lesion, with extension of tenderness down the patellar tendon and palpable enlargement. These more serious tendon lesions can be confirmed by ultrasound, computerised tomography or nuclear magnetic resonance scanning and may require surgical intervention in athletes in particular.

The *inferior patellar attachment* should be injected (Fig. 9.20) by accurately localising the maximal point of tenderness and then by directing the needle, after insertion, just to the side of the tendon, at an angle of about 45°, with the

with one finger (Fig. 9.22). A tender *medial plica*, which can be rolled under the finger at about the midpoint of the

Fig. 9.22 Method of palpation for localised medial patellar tenderness before local injection. Arrow indicates site of medial patella plica.

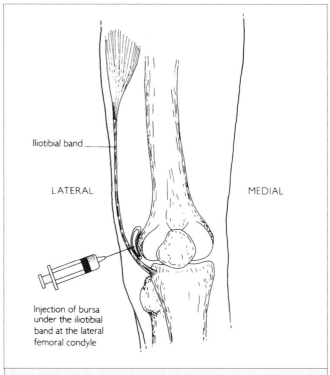

Fig. 9.23 Injection of the iliotibial band syndrome

knee extended so that the posterior attachment is infiltrated together with the paratendon as the needle is withdrawn. About 5 days after injection a graduated restrengthening programme of quadriceps exercises must be followed as full recovery of tendon strength takes many months.

Iliotibial band (ITB) syndrome

Pain due to this syndrome is typically felt after running about 7 miles, settles with rest, but then recurs after running a similar distance. Examination reveals local tenderness and ITB tightness (Ober's test, p. 93). Exclude leg length inequality or hyperpronation of the foot as the underlying mechanism (see p. 138) Injection should be directed towards the most tender site, which is most commonly where the iliotibial band slips backwards and forwards over the lateral femoral condyle as the knee flexes and extends, particularly in distance road runners (especially camber running). There may be swelling due to a bursitis under the iliotibial band, which should be injected (Fig. 9.23).

10

The foot and ankle

The foot and ankle are specially designed to transmit body weight. The joints are capable of adjusting to cope with various terrains and the thick heel and toe pads are designed as 'shock absorbers'. In addition to being targets for systemic arthropathies, because of concentrated stresses, the foot and ankle often develop static deformities.

ANATOMY

The foot comprises 26 bones, a variable number of sesamoids, held together by multiple ligaments and 38 muscles. It has three functional units: the hindfoot comprising the calcaneum and talus; the midfoot comprising five small tarsal bones; and the forefoot consisting of the metatarsals and phalanges.

The joints (Figs 10.1 and 10.2)

The distal tibiofibular joint

This is a fibrous joint which allows slight separation during ankle dorsiflexion. It is strengthened by anterior and posterior ligaments and a deep transverse tibiofibular ligament.

The ankle joint

The ankle joint comprises three articulations—the tibiotalar (talocrural) joint, the subtalar joint and the talonavicular joint. The tibiotalar joint is a hinge joint between the distal tibia and fibula and the domed trochlea of the talus. The medial and lateral malleoli project distally to form a mortise that holds the talus, preventing rotation or lateral flexion. The tibia forms the weight-bearing portion of the ankle joint and the axis of movement passes through the malleoli. The trochlea of the talus is wider anteriorly than posteriorly. Therefore the ankle is more stable in dorsiflexion, as in

Fig. 10.1 The bony anatomy of the foot and ankle—lateral aspect.

Fig. 10.2 The bony anatomy of the foot and ankle—medial aspect.

ascending inclines, than in plantar flexion, as in descending inclines. The joint capsule is attached around the articular margins of the tibia, fibula and talus. It is lax and weak on the anterior and posterior aspects of the ankle and anteriorly it is particularly extensive, extending from the tibia to a point approximately 1 cm distal to the neck of the talus. The capsule is lined by synovium and the articular cavity does not communicate with other joints or bursae. At the sides, the joint is strengthened by collateral ligaments (Fig. 10.3). The lateral collateral ligament is in three distinct bands, each of which can be separately damaged in a sprain injury. The medial (deltoid) ligament is triangular shaped, joining the medial malleolus to the talus, navicular and calcaneum. It is stronger than the lateral ligament and during eversion injury, rather than ligament rupture, the medial malleolus is fractured. The *subtalar (talocalcaneal) joint* is between the concave facet on the upper surface of the talus and the posterior convex facet on the upper surface of the calcaneum. It is sometimes known as the posterior subtalar joint. It permits inversion and eversion of the foot allowing one to stand upright on a sloping surface.

The *mid-tarsal joint* is a composite formed by the *talocalcaneo-navicular* joint and the *calcaneocuboid* joint. It allows the forefoot to invert (supinate) and evert (pronate) on the midfoot and other intertarsal joints and the tarsometatarsal joints add to the movement. The *talocalcaneo-navicular joint* is a ball-and-socket joint between the head of the talus and a socket formed by the concave posterior surface of the navicular and anterior facet in the upper surface of the calcaneum (sometimes known as the anterior subtalar joint).

The metatarsophalangeal (MTP) joints and interphalangeal joints

These are ellipsoid joints similar to the metacarpophalangeal joints of the hand. Each joint has a thick plantar (volar) plate, the plates being connected by the deep transverse metatarsal ligament. Two sesamoid bones are embedded into the volar plate beneath the hallux. The joints are flexed by the intrinsic muscles of the foot, while the extensor hallucis longus and extensor digitorum longus and brevis are dorsiflexors. The first metatarsophalangeal joint has a particularly important role in normal gait. For the hallux to function properly it needs 60–70° of dorsiflexion at the MTP joint, and disorders that limit this, such as hallux valgus and hallux rigidus, interfere with gait (especially 'toe-off' phase) as a consequence.

The interphalangeal joints are hinge joints which flex during the push-off phase of gait. In addition to helping to provide leverage for propelling the body forwards, the toes also provide stability and balance in both standing and movement by their gripping action on the ground.

The arch of the foot

This enables the weight of the body to be equally distributed between the posterior part of the calcaneum, which forms the prominence of the heel, and the heads of the four metatarsals and the two sesamoids of the first metatarsal anteriorly. The basic structure of the arch, which has a longitudinal and transverse component, is provided by the shape of the small bones of the foot united by many articular joints and supported by ligaments and muscles to provide flexibility and spring to facilitate walking and running.

The longitudinal arch is high and flexible on the medial side where it is formed by the medial three metatarsals, cuneiforms, navicula, talus and calcaneum. It is supported by several layers of ligaments (Fig. 10.4). Deepest is the strong spring ligament (plantar calcaneonavicular ligament), a broad thick band which connects the medial projection of the calcaneum (sustentaculum tali) to the navicula. The long and short plantar ligaments then join the calcaneum to the metatarsal bones and the cuboid. The most superficial layer is the plantar fascia which extends from the posterior inferior surface of the calcaneum to the transverse metatarsal ligament and the flexor tendon sheath of the toes, and acts as a strong tie between the weight-bearing points of the foot. The lateral side of the longitudinal arch is low and

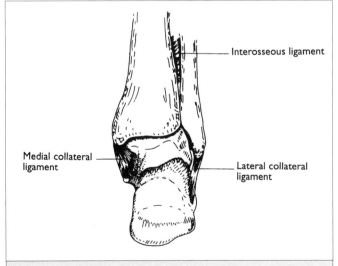

Fig. 10.3 Major ligaments of the ankle (talocrural) joint.

Interosseous ligament

Medial collateral ligament

Lateral collateral ligament

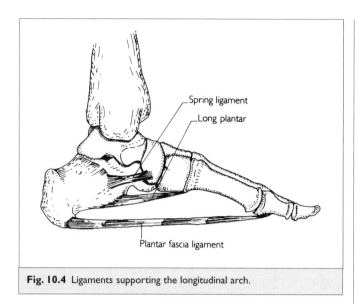

Fig. 10.4 Ligaments supporting the longitudinal arch.

rigid. The transverse arch is highest proximally across the cuboid and cuneiforms, and low distally across the metatarsal necks.

Tendons and bursae

The extrinsic muscles of the foot and ankle form three compartments in the lower leg. The anterior compartment contains the dorsiflexors of the foot and ankle; the lateral compartment contains the peroneal muscles, which act as plantar flexors and abductors; and the posterior compartment contains the plantar flexors. Anterior to the ankle are three tendon sheaths held in place by the extensor retinaculum (Fig. 10.5). This consists of a superior part (transverse crural ligament) in the anterior and inferior portion of the leg and an inferior part (cruciate ligament) in the proximal portion of the dorsum of the foot. The medial tendon sheath contains the tibialis anterior; the central sheath contains the extensor hallucis longus, extensor digitorum and peroneus tertius. Behind and below the lateral malleolus are the peroneus longus and brevis held down by the peroneal retinaculum, which consists of a superior and an inferior part.

Behind and below the medial malleolus are the tendons of the tibialis posterior, flexor digitorum longus and flexor hallucis longus, each in a tendon sheath (Fig. 10.6). These are held in place by the flexor retinaculum. Posteriorly the Achilles tendon (tendon calcaneus), the common tendon of the gastrocnemius and soleus, is inserted into the posterior aspect of the calcaneus. There are bursae between the skin and the Achilles tendon (retroachilles bursa) and between the tendon and the calcaneus (retrocalcaneal bursa) (Fig.

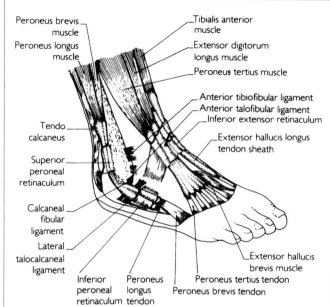

Fig. 10.5 Major tendons and tendon sheaths on lateral aspect of the ankle and foot.

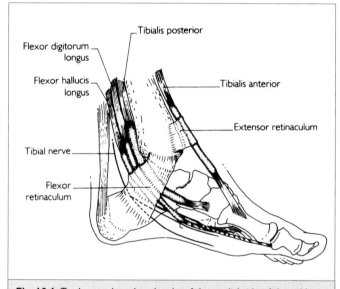

Fig. 10.6 Tendons and tendon sheaths of the medial side of the ankle.

10.7). At the plantar aspect of the midcalcaneum is the subcalcaneal bursa. There is also a small bursa anterior to the medial and lateral malleolus.

The tarsal tunnel lies between the medial malleolus and the calcaneus, roofed by the flexor retinaculum. In addition to tendons, the posterior tibial nerve passes through the tunnel.

Fig. 10.7 Bursae around the ankle.

Retroachilles bursa

Retrocalcaneal bursa

Subcalcaneal bursa

Plantar aponeurosis

Fig. 10.9 An abnormally high arch (pes cavus).

DEVELOPMENT

Lower limb buds first appear at about the fourth week of embryonic life. By 6–8 weeks proximal and distal segments are apparent and toes begin differentiation. Cartilaginous precursors of future bones develop. Bones of the foot are still largely cartilaginous at birth and are still deformable. Ossification occurs throughout the first 3 years and fusion of the phalangeal and metatarsal epiphyses is complete by late adolescence. The arch of the foot does not appear until approximately the third year and can be delayed until adolescence.

Developmental abnormalities

Clubfoot (talipes) is a deformity of the ankle and foot (Fig. 10.8). There may be plantar flexion of the ankle (talipes equinus) or dorsiflexion (talipes calcaneus). Often there is an

Fig. 10.8 Talipes equinus (left) and calcaneus (right).

associated midfoot deformity, for example, talipes equinovarus or talipes calcaneovalgus.

Flat foot (pes planus) is where there is absence of a longitudinal arch. This may be associated with a valgus deformity of the midfoot. *Pes cavus* is the opposite (Fig. 10.9) and is often associated with a varus deformity. Abnormal fibrous, bony or cartilaginous connections between the bones of the hind- and midfoot result in tarsal coalition. It often results in a painful, pronated gait because of lack of movement between the involved bones, with spasm of adjacent muscles.

The metatarsals may be adducted. Involvement of the first metatarsal (*metatarsus primus varus*) is most common and may precede hallux valgus deformity. Toes may be shortened (*brachydactyly*), fused (*syndactyly*), decreased in number (*hypodactyly*), absent (*adactyly*) or there may be extra toes (*polydactyly*).

SYMPTOMS

Pain is the principal symptom. In synovitis, pain is often diffuse and accompanied by prolonged stiffness, typically in the mornings. When due to static deformities, osteoarthritis and metatarsalgia, pain is more obviously associated with weight-bearing. Pain from the talocrural and the subtalar joints arises from the ankle and is aggravated by standing or walking, particularly on uneven terrain in the case of the subtalar joints. With the midtarsal joints pain is felt midway down the foot, while in the case of the MTP joints there is a characteristic sensation of 'walking on marbles', with pain localised to the metatarsal heads. Burning pain in the soles and toes may be caused by plantar neuralgia, Morton's neuroma (which often causes burning pain between the 3rd and 4th digits) and a tarsal tunnel syndrome.

The innervation of the foot is shown in Figure 10.10. The spine and all the other lower extremity joints should be

Fig. 10.10 Innervation of the foot and ankle.

examined, since pathology of these sites can be the cause of pain referred to the foot and ankle.

Referred pain from irritation of the first sacral nerve root affects the heel and the lateral side of the foot, is exacerbated by straight-leg raising, and may be accompanied by other neurological signs.

The most common causes of heel pain are Achilles tendinitis, retrocalcaneal bursitis and plantar fasciitis. Achilles tendinitis causes pain during the push-off phase of walking. Retrocalcaneal bursitis causes posterior heel pain aggravated by dorsiflexion of the ankle. Plantar fasciitis produces localised pain on the under-surface of the heel on weight-bearing. Sudden painful loss of the medial arch, particularly in runners, suggests rupture of tibialis posterior tendon. Recurrent pain and swelling after ankle inversion injury, with talar dome tenderness, points to osteochondral damage requiring imaging for confirmation.

Tarsal tunnel syndrome

This is caused by entrapment of the posterior tibial nerve beneath the flexor retinaculum behind and under the medial malleolus. Symptoms of burning, tingling and numbness can be felt throughout the distribution of the posterior tibial nerve but is often most pronounced in the toes and the dis-

tal part of the sole and may be more prominent at night. Often there is tenderness along the nerve at the margin of the medial malleolus, and there may be the equivalent of a Tinel's sign with percussion over the flexor retinaculum. Sometimes there is reduced pin-prick sensation but motor weakness and atrophy of the toe flexors and abductor hallucis is not common. Neurophysiological tests may demonstrate prolonged nerve conduction distal to the compression.

EXAMINATION

Inspection

Examination of the foot and ankle must include inspection of the whole lower limb and therefore the patient should remove clothing from the waist down. The ankle and foot are inspected both resting and standing, together with the footwear, which can provide important clues. Both sides are compared from all angles for swelling, deformities, the location of calluses and bursal reactions, the presence of other cutaneous manifestations and the appearance of the nails.

Inflammation producing capsular distension of the ankle joint produces diffuse swelling anteriorly, which obliterates the small depressions normally present in front of the malleoli. Sometimes there is swelling in the area of the tarsal tunnel just posterior to the joint between the malleoli and the Achilles tendon. Swelling of the ankle may be accentuated by dorsiflexion and inversion of the foot, which produces bulging beneath the extensor tendons in front of the lateral and medial malleolar ligaments.

Capsular distension of the midtarsal joint is less common but can produce diffuse swelling over the dorsum of the hindfoot. The MTP joints, however, frequently become swollen, being apparent in the dorsum of the forefoot and obscuring the visibility of the extensor tendons. Associated inflammation of ligaments bracing the forefoot results in spreading the metatarsals and toes.

Tenosynovitis of ankle extensors produces linear swelling across the ankle joint. Digital flexor tenosynovitis produces 'sausage' toes, which are characteristic of psoriatic arthritis.

In oedematous states, fluid collects below and behind the malleoli where tissues are most lax, producing swelling that pits.

In pes planus or flat foot there is loss of the longitudinal arch. In extreme cases the translocated talus and navicular produce a prominence in front of and slightly below the medial malleolus. The converse is pes cavus, which is usually congenital but may be the result of neurological disease such as spina bifida and cerebellar ataxia. Fixed plantar flexion of the foot (talipes equinus) is usually the result of spastic paralysis but can occur in rheumatoid arthritis as a result of shortening of the Achilles tendon. Deformities of the subtalar joint, calcaneovalgus (eversion) or calcaneovarus (inversion) are best observed from the back.

The commonest deformity of the big toe is hallux valgus (Fig. 10.11). There is lateral deviation of the big toe as a result of abnormal angulation and rotation of the first MTP joint. The first metatarsal deviates medially, resulting in increased width of the forefoot. Frequently there is a bursal reaction resulting in a bunion over the medial aspect of the joint. A hammer toe deformity (Fig. 10.12) results from hyperexten-

sion of the MTP joint, flexion of the proximal interphalangeal joint (PIP) and hyperextension of the distal interphalangeal joint (DIP). A callus often develops over the prominent PIP joint. The second toe is most often affected and this is frequently associated with hallux valgus of the big toe. This may occur with or without arthritis as an underlying cause. Sometimes the DIP is in a neutral position so that the tip of the toe touches the floor. This is a 'mallet toe'.

Cock-up (or claw) toe deformities (Fig. 10.13) are the result of flexion of the interphalangeal joints secondary to plantar subluxation of the MTP joints. There is often callus formation on the sole over the metatarsal heads and metatarsal spread due to weakening of the transverse metatarsal ligament. This is associated with a polyarthritis such as rheumatoid arthritis. Severe articular damage of the interphalangeal joints results in hyperextension deformities of the toes. Also, there can be lateral displacement of the proximal phalanges on the metatarsal head of all the toes, equivalent to 'ulnar deviation' of the fingers, leading to overlapping of the toes (Figs 10.14 and 10.15).

Abnormalities of gait may be observed. These include the toe-out gait, with outward displacement of the forefoot and an attempt to walk by rolling the foot from the lateral to the medial side. This happens in patients with painful ankles and often results in an eversion deformity and loss of the longitudinal arch so that the patient walks on the medial aspect of the foot. A toe-in gait (pigeon-toe) is due to inward displacement of the forefoot which is often congenital and associated with inversion of the foot. Those with a painful heel will not allow the heel to strike the ground, and a foot drop results in a typical 'slap' of the foot on the ground.

Fig. 10.11 Hallux valgus with spread of the forefoot.

Fig. 10.12 Hammer toe deformity.

Fig. 10.13 Claw toe deformity.

Fig. 10.14 Hallux valgus and cock-up toe deformities due to subluxation MTPs in rheumatoid arthritis.

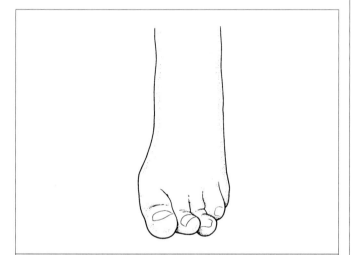

Fig. 10.15 Severe hyperextension deformities associated with subluxation of the interphalangeal joints due to rheumatoid arthritis, resulting in flailing toes.

When examining the shoes, a broken medial counter is typical of flat feet, excessive wear of the lateral border of the shoe is typical of hallux rigidus and scuffed toes occur in those with a dropped foot.

In addition to defining calluses, examination of the skin and nails may demonstrate psoriasis or other characteristic lesions such as keratoderma blenorrhagica. Dependent rubor indicates vascular disease.

Palpation

Examination is best facing the patient who sits on the edge of the couch with the legs dangling free. With one hand cup-

ping the heel to support the foot, the examiner palpates the anterior aspect of the ankle and forefoot with the fingers (Fig. 10.16) or thumb (Fig. 10.17) of the other hand. An alternative method is to support the foot with the fingers of both hands and use both thumbs to palpate the tissue anteriorly (Fig. 10.18). Since synovial reflection is most extensive over

Fig. 10.16 Palpation of the ankle. The patient's foot is supported by the examiner's hand, which compresses the posterior aspect of the articular capsule. This distends the articular capsule and synovial membrane anteriorly, where they can be palpated by the fingers of the examiner's hand.

Fig. 10.17 Palpation of the ankle using the thumb.

Fig. 10.18 Alternative method of palpating the ankle.

Fig. 10.19 Pes planus—the talar head displaces medially and plantarward.

Fig. 10.20 Left: medial prominence of the head of the talus in pes planus. Right: callosity development over the head of the talus in association with shoe-wearing.

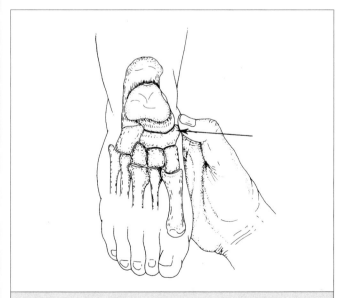

Fig. 10.21 The navicular tubercle (arrow).

the anterior aspect of the joint, synovial thickening or effusion is likely to be palpable anteriorly. Sometimes it is best palpated medially and laterally between the extensor retinaculum and malleoli. By compressing the area beneath and behind the medial and lateral malleoli with the supporting hand, thus compressing the posterior aspect of the articular capsule, the anterior capsule can be distended with synovial fluid. The anterior capsule is best palpated for tenderness over the joint line medial to the tendon of tibialis anterior (the most medial of the three extensor tendons). Tenosynovitis overlying the anterior aspect of the ankle joint can be distinguished from underlying synovitis by more superficial linear swelling and tenderness, which extends beyond the joint margin, over the distribution of the tendon sheaths. Pain produced by resisted movement of the affected tendon is also characteristic.

The subtalar joint is not accessible to palpation but the intertarsal joints can be palpated for swelling and tenderness, which is mainly detected in the dorsum of the foot. The head of the talus becomes prominent on the medial side of the foot in pes planus (Fig. 10.19), and there may be overlying tenderness and callus from pressing against the shoe (Fig. 10.20). In children there may be tenderness over the navicular tubercle as a result of osteochondritis of the os tibialis externa (os naviculare), often associated with sport (Fig. 10.21).

The MTP joints are palpated between the examiner's thumbs on the dorsum of the foot, and the forefinger on the plantar aspect over the metatarsal head. Each joint is examined individually for soft-tissue thickening, deformity and tenderness (Fig. 10.22). The medial aspect of the first MTP is a common site for a tender and inflamed bursa (Fig. 10.23). It is also a common site for tophi. In the presence of chronic synovitis, there is frequently subluxation of the MTP joints with dorsal displacement of the proximal phalanx and loss

Fig. 10.22 Palpation of metatarsophalangeal joints of the foot. Left: plantar view. Right: lateral view. The forefinger is palpating deeply between the second and third metatarsal head.

Fig. 10.23 The medial aspect of the first MTP is a common site for an inflamed bursa.

of the normal fat pad under the metatarsal bones so that the metatarsal heads are easily palpated. Synovial proliferation and joint effusion can be palpated as soft-tissue thickening partially obliterating the grooves between adjacent metatarsal heads. Sometimes tenderness over specific joints cannot be elicited but this important sign of synovitis may be obtained by grasping the forefoot and squeezing the metatarsal heads together between the thumb on one side of the foot and the fingers on the other (the metatarsal compression test—Fig. 10.24).

Sharply localised tenderness between the 3rd and 4th (less commonly between the 2nd and 3rd) metatarsal heads is characteristic of Morton's interdigital neuroma. Tenderness may be accompanied by altered sensation on the lateral and medial aspects of the 3rd and 4th toes, respectively and, very occasionally, a large interdigital neuroma may be palpated. There is often a click on cross compression. Localised tenderness over the dorsum of the 2nd or 3rd metatarsal (although any metatarsal can be involved) may indicate a 'march' fracture. Localised tenderness under an MTP joint (especially 1st) may be due to sesamoiditis (particularly the medial sesamoid).

The thumb and forefinger are used to palpate the interphalangeal joints of the toes. Swelling and tenderness due to synovitis are most prominent on the medial and lateral aspects of the joint. The Achilles tendon is palpated between thumb and forefinger for swelling, tenderness and the presence of nodules such as rheumatoid nodules, xanthomata or tophi. Repeated microtearing may lead to degeneration of the tendon, referred to as tendonosis (see p. 126). There are both local and systemic causes of tendinitis or paratendinitis of

Fig. 10.24 Metatarsal compression test.

Fig. 10.25 Palpation of the Achilles tendon (left) and calcaneal bursa (right).

the Achilles tendon, and these may also cause inflammation of related structures. The calcaneal bursa, for example, lying between the skin and the insertion of the Achilles tendon, is particularly subject to local trauma (Fig. 10.25). On the other hand, inflammation of the deeper retrocalcaneal bursa between the calcaneus and the Achilles tendon may signify inflammation with a systemic cause. After rupture of the Achilles tendon, a defect may be palpable. To test the continuity of the tendon, the patient lies prone on the couch. On squeezing the calf, the normal plantar flexion of the foot is greatly reduced or absent after rupture of the tendon (Fig. 10.26).

The plantar surface of the foot should be smooth and non-tender. Tenderness on the sole near the heel may indicate plantar fasciitis, which may be the result of local trauma or part of a systemic disorder. Sometimes the tenderness arises from soft tissues overlying a bony spur on the plantar surface of the calcaneum, near the site of attachment of the plantar fascia (Fig. 10.27).

Range of movements

Figure 10.28 illustrates techniques to screen for gross restriction of ankle and foot movement. These should be followed by more detailed examination of the passive range of movements.

Fig. 10.26 Testing for continuity of the gastrocnemius and soleus muscles' common tendon. Absence of plantar flexion of the foot indicates a ruptured Achilles tendon.

Ankles

Movements should be tested with the knees flexed and the legs dangling to relax the gastrocnemius. Stabilise the subtalar joint by grasping the calcaneum and avoid forefoot movement by inverting the forefoot and pushing the foot as

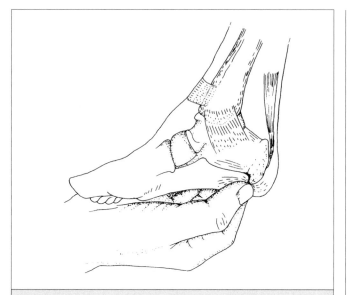

Fig. 10.27 Testing for tenderness over the site of attachment of the plantar fascia.

Restricted movement may also be due to periarticular oedema from various causes and contraction of the joint capsule and periarticular tissues.

To examine movements of the subtalar joint, stabilise the distal leg with one hand and grasp the heel with the other to move the foot into inversion and eversion (Fig. 10.30). Movement of the midtarsal joint is tested by holding the calcaneum in one hand and rotating the foot with the other in the plane of the sole of the foot (Fig. 10.31, showing 30° inversion and 40° eversion). Figure 10.32 shows the range of flexion and extension in the 1st MTP. The other MTP joints have approximately 40° of flexion and extension. The PIP joints flex to approximately 50° and the DIPs to approximately 40°, with a varying degree of extension up to 30°.

Tests of stability

The anterior drawer signs tests the integrity of the anterior talofibular ligament (Fig. 10.33). Placing one hand on the anterior aspect of the lower tibia, the examiner grasps the calcaneum with the other hand and draws the calcaneum and talus anteriorly while pushing the tibia posteriorly.

one unit with the examiner's other hand into dorsiflexion and plantar flexion (Fig. 10.29). In the damaged joint the movement is restricted, painful and often accompanied by crepitus. In synovitis, the range is restricted and the extremes of dorsiflexion and plantar flexion are painful.

Fig. 10.28 Quick tests for foot and ankle range of motion.

Fig. 10.29 Testing ankle dorsiflexion (left) and plantar flexion (right).

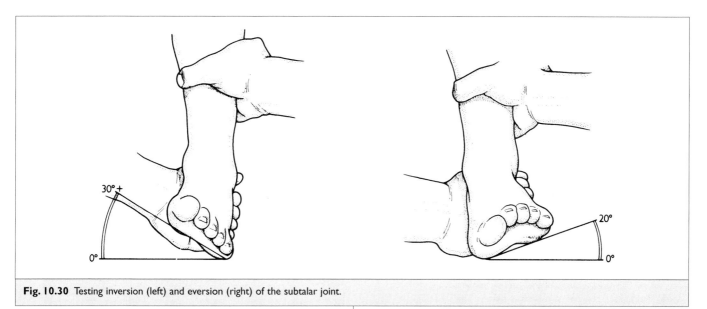

Fig. 10.30 Testing inversion (left) and eversion (right) of the subtalar joint.

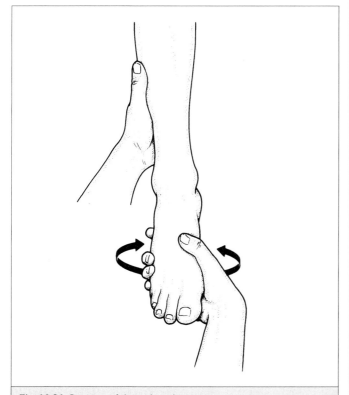

Fig. 10.31 Rotation of the midtarsal joint.

Fig. 10.32 The range of flexion and extension in the 1st MTP.

Fig. 10.33 The anterior drawer sign tests the anterior talofibular ligament. Movement indicates a tear of the ligament.

Movement, which is normally not present, indicates tear of the ligament, usually as a result of a severe sprain. To test for lateral instability, which results from damage to both the anterior talofibular ligament and the calcaneofibular ligament, invert the calcaneum. On the lateral side a 'gap' appears between the talus and the calcaneum (Fig. 10.34). For deltoid ligament insufficiency the calcaneum is everted and a gap develops between the talus and calcaneum.

Fig. 10.34 Evaluating stability of the anterior talofibular and calcaneofibular ligaments: if they are torn, the ankle is unstable.

Muscle testing (Table 10.1)

Plantar flexion. Unless there is major foot deformity, inability of the patient to walk on toes indicates significant muscle weakness. Gross muscle weakness can also be assessed when the patient lies supine with legs extended and a pad under the knees to prevent hyperextension. Stabilising the lower leg with one hand, the examiner's other hand provides graded resistance to plantar flexion (Fig. 10.35).

Dorsiflexion and inversion. If the patient can walk on his or her heels, muscle strength is considered normal. Alternatively, test the tibialis anterior with the patient sitting, using one hand to stabilise the lower leg and the other to provide resistance to flexion and inversion (Fig. 10.36).

Fig. 10.35 Test for plantar flexors.

Table 10.1. Nerve roots, peripheral nerves and muscles involved in movement of the ankle and foot

Movement	Nerve root	Peripheral nerve	Muscles
Plantar flexion	S1, S2	Tibial	Gastrocnemius, soleus (accessory muscles: tibialis posterior, peroneus longus and brevis, flexor hallucis longus, flexor digitorum longus, plantaris)
Dorsiflexion and inversion	L4, L5	Deep peroneal	Tibialis anterior
Inversion (in plantar flexion)	L5, S1	Tibial	Tibialis posterior
Eversion	S1	Superficial peroneal	Peroneus longus and brevis
Flexion of big toe			
MTP joint	L4, L5, S1	Medial plantar	Flexor hallucis brevis
IP joint	L5, S1, S2	Tibial nerve	Flexor hallucis longus
Extension of big toe			
MTP joint	L5, S1	Deep peroneal	Extensor digitorum brevis
IP joint	L4, L5, S1	Deep peroneal	Extensor hallucis longus
Flexion of toes 2–5			
MTP joint	L4, L5	Medial (1st lumbrical)	Lumbricals
	S1, S2	Lateral (2nd to 4th lumbricals) plantar	
PIP joint	L4, L5	Medial plantar	Flexor digitorum brevis
DIP joint	L5, S1	Tibial	Flexor digitorum longus
Extension of toes 2–5	L4, L5, S1	Deep peroneal	Extensor digitorum longus
	L5, S1	Deep peroneal	Extensor digitorum brevis

Eversion of the foot. If the patient is able to walk on the medial borders of the feet, muscle strength is normal. It can be tested manually by stabilising the foot and resisting plantar flexion and eversion by pushing against the lateral border of the foot (Fig. 10.37).

Inversion of the foot. The tibialis posterior is tested by stabilising the lower leg with one hand and having the patient plantar flex and invert the foot while the examiner resists this movement with the other hand.

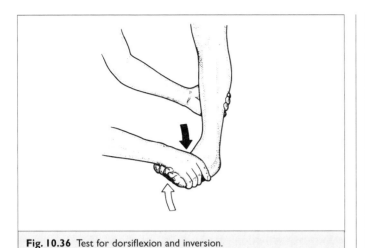

Fig. 10.36 Test for dorsiflexion and inversion.

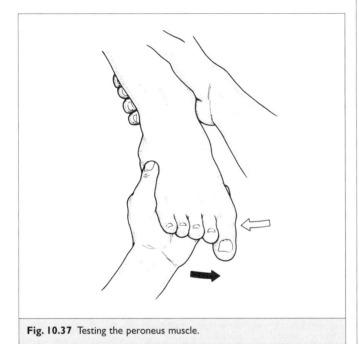

Fig. 10.37 Testing the peroneus muscle.

Fig. 10.38 Testing the flexors of the 2nd to 5th toes.

Flexion and extension of the toes. To test flexion and extension of the big toe, the foot is stabilised with one hand in the midtarsal region and flexion at the MTP and the IP joints are assessed against resistance provided by the examiner's other hand placed beneath the proximal phalanx. Extension is tested against resistance of the examiner's thumb on the nailbed with fingers on the ball of the foot to stabilise the metatarsal. To test the extensor hallucis longus, resistance must be applied distal to the IP joint.

To test the flexors of the other toes, the patient flexes these joints against resistance provided by the examiner's fingers, which are beneath the proximal row of phalanges (Fig. 10.38). The MT and IP joints should be unyielding.

To test extension of the toes, the calcaneum is held to stabilise the foot and resistance to movement is provided by the thumb of the examiner's other hand on the dorsum of the toes. These should be unyielding.

LOCAL ASPIRATION AND INJECTION

The ankle joint

There are several approaches to aspirating and injecting the ankle joint. The anterior approach is described here. Injection of the ankle joint is more liable to be complicated by infection than other sites, perhaps because of the tendency to oedema. Therefore a careful aseptic technique is particularly important.

With the foot in moderate plantar flexion, insert the needle in the space between the tibia and talus bounded medially by the tibialis anterior tendon and laterally by extensor hallucis longus tendon (Fig. 10.39). It is important to direct the needle tangentially to the curve of the talus; the most common mistake is to direct the needle too much towards the heel.

Posterior subtalar joint

This often communicates with the ankle joint, particularly in rheumatoid arthritis. Therefore injection specifically into

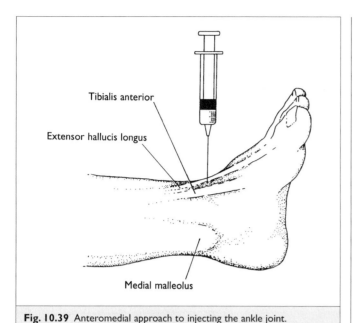

Fig. 10.39 Anteromedial approach to injecting the ankle joint.

this joint, which can be difficult, is not often needed. The joint can be injected using a lateral approach with the patient lying prone. The landmarks (Fig. 10.40) are a horizontal line drawn 2.5 cm above the distal end of the lateral malleolus, and a vertical line 1.0 cm from the posterior border of the shaft of the fibula. The point where these lines cross marks the site of entry.

Midtarsal joint

Injection is difficult. Sometimes a small-gauge needle can be inserted into an intertarsal joint space on the dorsum of the foot.

First metatarsophalangeal joint

Locate and mark the superolateral joint line on the lateral side. The joint is aspirated and injected through the dorsum of the toe with the needle entering tangentially from the lateral side (Fig. 10.41).

Achilles bursitis

Approach from the lateral side of the heel, just above the top of the calcaneum. Direct the needle medially and downwards into the bursa, which lies just beneath the skin. Avoid injecting the tendon *per se*.

Achilles tendinitis/peritendinitis

Achilles pain and tendon enlargement in athletes should be assessed in the relaxed position, and then tension applied by dorsiflexion of the foot. Pain induced by finger pressure on the relaxed tendon, which disappears on repeat pressure at the same site when the tendon is put under full stretch, suggests a deep tendon lesion (tendonosis or tendon degeneration, usually due to repeated microtearing, particularly at the vulnerable watershed area of the tendon). If the pain induced by finger pressure is the same relaxed as under stretch, paratendinitis is likely to be present; if paratendinitis alone, the swelling is usually less and more focal. However, assessment by imaging (ultrasound, MRI or CT scan) is advisable before a peritendinous injection is given. Where there is no significant tendonosis on scan, paratendon injection appears safe, if followed by a short period of rest and then a carefully graduated restrengthening programme.

Fig. 10.40 Injection of the posterior subtalar joint.

Fig. 10.41 Injection of the first MTP joint.

Plantar fasciitis

Locate the site of maximum tenderness on the plantar surface of the heel. The needle can be inserted through the plantar surface or alternatively using a medial approach. Here, the needle is inserted through the thinner skin on the medial side of the heel so that the point lies beneath the tender spot, and the injection is made as close as possible to the bony surface into the tendinuous insertion.

Morton's neuroma

Palpate for the point of maximum tenderness and inject.

Tenosynovitis of posterior tibial tendon

Often the tendon sheath is swollen. A tangential approach is used, directing the needle proximally. A correctly placed injection distends the tendon sheath further.

A similar procedure is used for the peroneal tendon sheaths posterior to the lateral malleolus.

Tarsal tunnel syndrome

Inject under the flexor retinaculum between the calcaneum and the medial malleolus.

11

The temporomandibular joint

The articulation between mandible and cranium consists of components that are concerned with mastication, swallowing, speech and respiration, as well as mandibular posture. Disorders affecting the temporomandibular joints may be congenital, or arise from disease, degenerative processes, trauma or as a concomitant of occlusal stress and muscle spasm.

ANATOMY

The temporomandibular joints are unique; the mandible connects the two joints so that they move in unison—one joint cannot move alone. They are also the only joints whose movement is linked and guided by the dental occlusion; therefore tooth loss or dental restoration may affect the joints.

The primary components of the temporomandibular joint are the mandibular condyle, the articular surfaces of the temporal bone, the articular disc and the joint capsule (Fig. 11.1). The superior portion of the lateral pterygoid muscle is considered by some to be part of the joint because the disc is a direct extension of it; the inferior portion of the muscle attaches to the condyle. The temporomandibular joint contrasts with other joints in that its articular surfaces are fibrocartilage instead of hyaline cartilage.

The disc is a dense fibrous plate that separates the joints into superior and inferior compartments. It is characterised by a thin, avascular central portion and a thicker, vascular posterior portion. The meniscus is closely moulded to the mandibular condyle and the lower joint compartment is small and difficult to enter. The disc is normally tightly bound to the medial and lateral poles of the condyle and its main functions are stabilisation during condylar movement and shock absorption during mastication. The joint capsule attaches to the articular eminence of the temporal bone and

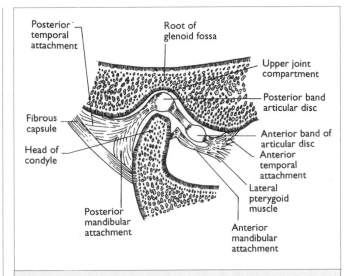

Fig. 11.1 Anatomy of the temporomandibular joint. The meniscus divides the joint into an upper and lower portion.

to the condyle. The capsule is reinforced on the lateral aspect by the temporomandibular ligament, which provides some limitation to mandibular movement, and medially by the sphenomandibular ligament. The articular eminence, not the glenoid fossa, is the primary functional area of the temporal bone during mandibular movements.

The two condylar movements during mandibular function are rotation and translation. In normal active opening of the mouth there is a combination of hinge and gliding movement. The superior joint space is associated with the anterior gliding movements of translation, whereas the inferior joint surface is associated with condylar rotation (Fig. 11.2). Because both temporomandibular joints are joined by a single bone, movement in one joint cannot occur without either similar coordinating or dissimilar reactive movements in the other joints. Opening, closing, protrusion and restriction are bilateral symmetrical movements. Lateral excursions are bilateral asymmetrical movements.

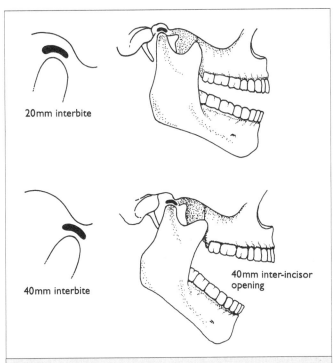

Fig. 11.2 The hinge and glide motions of the temporomandibular joint in an open position.

Mandibular opening is produced by contraction of the lateral pterygoid muscles with assistance from the digastric, geniohyoid and myohyoid muscles. The masseter, medial pterygoid and anterior fibres of the temporalis muscles are involved in mandibular closing. Protrusion of the mandible is achieved by the lateral pterygoid muscles, whereas the retruded position is produced by contraction of the posterior fibres of the temporalis muscles. Sideward movement of the mandible occurs when the contralateral lateral pterygoid muscle contracts.

The temporalis muscle plays a major role in the limitation of joint loading, and the lateral pterygoid muscle helps to stabilise the joint by controlling both the meniscus (upper head of lateral pterygoid) and the condylar position (lower head of lateral pterygoid muscle).

The major sensory innervation of the temporomandibular joint is derived from branches of the auriculotemporal nerve, with branches of the masseteric and posterior deep temporal nerves making a smaller contribution. The capsule, lateral ligament and posterior fat pads are innervated. However, the central part of the meniscus and the synovium do not appear to be innervated.

The superficial temporal artery is the primary blood supply to the joint.

FUNCTIONAL ANATOMY

The hinge movement of the lower joint allows some 40-mm of opening between the incisors and is seldom affected by joint dysfunction. Functional problems are usually related to the gliding or translatory movement of the upper joint space as the condyle moves forwards and down the articular eminence when the mouth opens. Restriction of opening may be a result of muscle spasm or displacement of the meniscus, which may or may not be reversible (Fig. 11.3).

The joint is non-load-bearing but appears to be load-bearing in some instances. This may be of importance as a cause of pain. The temporalis muscle has horizontal fibres that limit joint-loading. The aim of the conservative management of the joint (occlusal bite guards) is to reduce joint-loading and to keep the meniscus in the correct relationship to the condyle, thus restoring the dental occlusion and correcting the closing pathway determined by the interdigitation of the teeth.

PHYLOGENETIC DEVELOPMENT

The mammalian jaw joint is formed from membranous bones derived from the first branchial arch and cranium. In contrast, the jaw joint of most non-mammals ossifies from cartilaginous elements of the first branchial arch and its maxillary process. These primordial elements remain in the mammalian skull, but are in ossified form as the middle ear

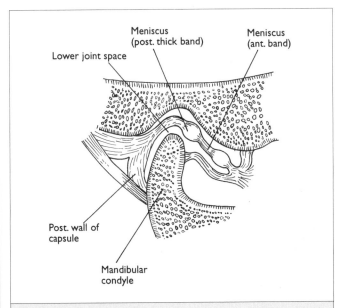

Fig. 11.3 Limited opening of the temporomandibular joint showing anterior displacement of the meniscus.

structures, malleus and incus. The articular disc, which characterises the mammalian joint, is a recent phylogenetic development.

DEVELOPMENTAL ABNORMALITIES

The condylar cartilage is a major mandibular growth centre, and therefore disease of the temporomandibular joint in childhood can affect mandibular development.

Familial traits of bilateral retrognathism or prognathism are not uncommon; bilateral temporomandibular maldevelopment (Treacher Collins syndrome) is very rare. Agenesis, hypoplasia or hyperplasia of the mandibular condyles, in the absence of other local or systemic anomalies, are uncommon. Severe otitis media, trauma and arthritis are the main acquired causes of impaired condylar development.

Impaired condylar growth is primarily characterised by a gradual deviation of the chin towards the affected side of the jaw and over-eruption of teeth on the non-affected side. Bilateral involvement can cause a retrognathic 'bird-like' facial profile.

In condylar hyperplasia, there is notable bony enlargement of the affected condyle and mandibular direction towards the contralateral side.

HISTORY

The specific points to elicit in the history are listed in Table 11.1.

The past medical history should always be reviewed. The patient should be questioned about previous illnesses, particularly rheumatoid arthritis and degenerative joint disease. It is important to note any trauma to the head and

Table 11.1. Important aspects of the history

- General/past history
  Previous consultations, e.g. ENT, dental
  Previous treatments
  Stress-related problems
  —headaches
  —disturbed sleep

- Pain
  Onset, duration
  Location, character
  Provoking factors, e.g. heat/cold, chewing

- Joint
  Limitation of movement
  Stiffness
  Locking
  Joint noises
  Habits, e.g. bruxism, nail-biting

neck. Injuries to the side of the face and chin are often responsible for temporomandibular joint problems.

The patient's dental history should also be reviewed, particularly if it coincides with the onset of symptoms.

There are numerous associated problems seen in the temporomandibular pain syndrome and patients rarely associate these with the facial pain. Habits such as bruxism and nail-biting exacerbate the pain and muscle spasm. Stress-related problems are invariably present. Tension headache with a pressure sensation over the top of the head and down the neck may be a daily occurrence. The headache may respond to simple analgesia but the dull ache in the jaw continues. Pain in the neck, back and abdomen and an irritable colon may also be present. The sleep pattern may be disturbed and this may be marked if there is also depression.

SYMPTOMS

Pain

Pain from the temporomandibular joint is the second most common facial pain after toothache. The main features are pain associated with mandibular movement, often accompanied by limitation of movement. Pain can be either localised to the joint or referred to the head, neck and shoulders. The patient's description of the location, duration and characteristics of the pain greatly helps in distinguishing between disorders with similar symptoms and physical findings.

The location of the pain should be confirmed by asking the patient to indicate where it hurts. This often helps differentiate between a true joint problem, in which the patient usually localises the discomfort in the pretragus region, and a muscular discomfort. It is also important to note whether the pain is unilateral or bilateral.

Pain associated with myofascial pain dysfunction is most often described as being a dull, unilateral ache that is often worse on waking. Joint pain may be constant, dull or sharp, but there is usually increasing discomfort with increasing function, and it is pronounced after chewing hard foods. The pain is worse on waking owing to bruxism in many patients, but some find the pain worse at the end of the day.

Clicking

This symptom is not uncommon and may be described as 'popping' or 'snapping'; its character is quite different from crepitus, which is described as 'grating'. Clicking is usually bilateral to auscultation, but patients often think only one joint is affected. Clicking occurs at a specific point of jaw movement whereas crepitus is present throughout. Clicking may vary from day to day and be absent at times. A loss of clicking and limitation of movement indicates displacement of the meniscus. Clicking may also be eliminated by placing a spatula between the teeth simulating a bite guard.

Limitation of mandibular movement

The range of opening may be limited; this may be either constant or intermittent occurring only at the end or beginning of the day. The limitation takes the form of the jaw 'sticking' or 'locking'. Locking can vary in frequency and severity. It may occur at regular times of the day, the most common being on waking. It is sudden in onset and distressing. Patients use both terms when they have developed a way of 'freeing the joint'. This often takes the form of a lateral excursion or even pressing the mandible sideways with the hand. It may spontaneously resolve.

Locking may be a confusing term to the patient. They may describe this as jamming or dislocation of the joint. It usually occurs with the teeth slightly apart, during opening or closing of the mouth. Further movement is then prevented. Locking is the result of disc displacement. The range of movements is limited to rotational movements in the joint allowing opening to only 26 mm interincisorly, the translatory movement of the condyle and wide opening being prevented.

EXAMINATION

Inspection

Swelling of the joint must be moderate or marked before it is apparent. If swelling is detectable it appears as a rounded bulge in the area underlying the joint just anterior to the external auditory meatus.

The symmetry of the face should be assessed. Although mild to moderate asymmetry is common, gross asymmetry may reflect a growth disturbance of the joint which may have resulted from trauma in childhood. Hypertrophy of the masseter muscles may indicate clenching or other oral habits.

Note the rhythm of the opening and closing of the jaw. The mandible should open and close in a straight line, with the teeth coming together and separating easily. Pathology in one or both joints or an abnormal dentition will result in abnormality.

The meniscus divides the joint cavity in two portions, a lower part used for hinge motion and an upper portion used for gliding motion. On inspection of the temporomandibular joint the two motions can be observed, the joint hinges within the glenoid fossa and glides forward to the eminentia.

Palpation

The joint can be located by placing the top of the forefinger just anterior to the external auditory meatus. On opening the mouth the top of the finger drops into an area overlying the joint. Both pretragus depressions should be palpated simultaneously. The joint can also be palpated anteriorly in the external auditory canal (Fig. 11.4). In the presence of synovitis the joint may be swollen and tender.

It is important to assess during pretragus and intra-auricular palpation whether the condyles move symmetrically. When unilateral problems exist, the mandible will always be seen to deviate to the side with limited condylar movement. In addition to limitation of joint movement, palpation of these areas is also used to detect clicking and crepitus.

The regional muscles should be examined for tenderness and spasm. The temporalis, medial and lateral pterygoids, masseter, trapezius and sternocleidomastoid are the primary muscles included in the evaluation. The masseter muscles

Fig. 11.4 To palpate the temporomandibular joint, place index finger in the auditory canal, or over joint.

can be palpated bilaterally, with the fingers over the angle of the mandible. Tenderness should be detected at rest or when the jaw is clenched. The masseter muscles are most effectively examined by simultaneously pressing from inside and outside the mouth in a process of bimanual palpation.

The medial pterygoids are difficult to examine. They are checked by running a finger in an anteroposterior direction along the medial aspect of the mandible in the floor of the mouth. This can produce a gag reflex. The posterior border can be palpated extraorally by placing the fingers around the posterior border of the ramus of the mandible (Fig. 11.5).

The lateral pterygoid muscle is tested by placing a finger between the buccal mucosa and the superior gum and pointing the finger past the last upper molar to the neck of the mandible (Fig. 11.6). As the mouth opens, the neck of the mandible swings forward and the lateral pterygoid tightens. If the muscle has been damaged or is in spasm, the patient feels pain or tenderness. This muscle can also be examined by standing behind the patient, placing the palm of the hand over the chin and asking the patient to open gently against resistance and then to move the jaw laterally. This muscle has clinical importance, for if it is traumatised secondary to a stretch injury, it may go into spasm and cause temporomandibular joint pain, as well as asymmetrical sideways motion of the jaw.

To examine temporalis, palpate over the temporal area with the jaw relaxed and clenched. Remember that the muscle covers a wide area over the temple. The patient may well locate the area of tenderness.

The muscles of the neck and shoulder may also require examination. The ear should be examined auroscopically, if indicated, and the salivary glands palpated for swelling and tenderness.

Range of motion

Normally one can open the mouth wide enough to insert three fingers between the incisor teeth (c. 35–55 mm, normally greater than 40 mm; Fig. 11.7). Care should be taken to keep the lower jaw protruded during this measurement, because maximal opening of the mandible depends on adequate forward positioning of the lower jaw as well as on the degree of vertical motion. Note any deviation on opening or premature contacts.

Fig. 11.5 Palpation of the medial pterygoids.

Fig. 11.6 Palpation of the lateral pterygoid muscles.

Fig. 11.7 The normal mouth span is greater than 40 mm.

The temporomandibular joint also allows the jaw to glide forward or protrude. Normally it can protrude far enough for the bottom teeth to be in front of the upper teeth (usually more than 10 mm).

Lateral motion of the jaw is measured by partially opening the mouth, protruding the lower jaw, and then moving the lower jaw from side to side. Movement should be equal and in the region of 10 mm. It is best to evaluate lateral motion (normally 1–2 cm) with the jaw protruded as far as possible, as the position of the mandible in the anteroposterior direction can cause considerable variation in the degree of lateral motion of the jaw. Lateral movement is lost earlier and to a greater degree than vertical movement.

Limited opening or deviated mandibular movements are frequently seen on examination but patients are themselves often only aware of the limitation of opening. The temporomandibular pain syndrome is more often seen unilaterally, and the associated unilateral muscle spasm results in deviation of the mandible to the affected side. Deviation is clearly seen when the mouth is opened and viewed from the front.

Muscle and neurological examination

The muscles that close the mandible are the temporalis (deep temporal branches of the mandibular division of the facial nerve, C7), the masseter (masseteric nerve from the mandibular division of trigeminal nerve, C5) and the medial pterygoid (medial pterygoid nerve of the mandibular division of the trigeminal nerve). These muscles may be tested by forcing the closed mouth into an open position, and the size, firmness and strength of the temporalis and masseter muscles can be determined by palpation.

The muscles that open the mouth are the lateral pterygoid and the suprahyoid muscles. These consist of the digastric (mandibular division of the trigeminal nerve to the posterior belly and the facial nerve to the anterior belly), the mylohyoid (mandibular division of the trigeminal nerve), and the geniohyoid (hypoglossal nerve, C1). To test the muscles that open the mouth ask the patient to open against a resisting hand under the jaw. Normally they can open their mouth against maximum resistance. To test the pterygoids on the left side ask the patient to move the mandible forward and laterally to the right side against graded resistance, the examiner's hands being placed near the front of the mandible on the right side. Similarly, the right side muscles can be tested with the hand on the left side of the mandible.

Closure of the mouth is achieved by the masseter, temporalis and medial pterygoids. Ask the patient to resist an increasing opening force by placing a hand on the chin and supporting the forehead with the other hand. The *jaw reflex* is a stretch reflex involving the masseter and temporalis muscles. The 5th cranial (trigeminal) nerve innervates these muscles and mediates the reflex arc. Place a finger over the chin with the mouth slightly open; tapping the finger with a tendon hammer will elicit a reflex and close the mouth (Fig. 11.8).

Teeth and mouth

Note any carious teeth, restorations or dentures present. The attrition of teeth may indicate a grinding habit and a full occlusal analysis may be indicated.

Temporomandibular pain syndrome

This is also known by several other names, such as myofascial pain dysfunction. It can be defined as a chronic or acute musculoskeletal pain or dysfunction of the masticatory system, aggravated by jaw movement but independent of local oral or dental disease.

Fig. 11.8 Reflex tests—the jaw reflex.

It is most commonly seen in young people, being twice as common in women. It is usually a self-limiting condition with a time course of 3–9 months. The majority of patients respond to reassurance, but in 5% the pain is persistent and requires treatment.

ADDITIONAL TESTS

Investigations may be divided into those aiming to exclude causes of pain outside the joint complex and investigations of the joint itself.

Radiography

Conventional radiographs of the temporomandibular joint may not accurately reflect the joint components and their spatial relationships. These limitations may lead to an under-diagnosis of joint defects.

Tomography is superior as this can reproduce small changes in the central portion of the joint but this does expose the patient to more radiation. Computed tomography scanning and magnetic resonance imaging are increasingly being used.

Arthrography has assumed an important role in the diagnosis of the temporomandibular joint. Defects in the position or structure of the joint, disc and its attachments can be determined, and displacement or perforation of the disc, irregularities in the posterior attachment of the disc, and adhesions can be detected. The most common soft-tissue derangement of the joint has been shown in several studies using arthrography to be anterior disc placement.

Arthroscopy

Arthroscopic examination of the temporomandibular joint is increasingly being carried out. It is best performed under general anaesthesia, but may be performed under local anaesthesia with sedation. Only the upper joint space can be visualised. Internal derangement such as anterior displacement of the meniscus may be relieved by lysis and lavage of the joint.

Electromyography

One of the major criteria in diagnosing temporomandibular joint dysfunction is to find tenderness to palpation in one or more of the muscles of mastication and increased muscle activity. Electromyography provides an objective means of monitoring changes in muscle activity and is an important component of biofeedback treatment. Auditory or visual electromyographic feedback supplies information to the patient concerning muscle activity.

INJECTION TREATMENT

Painful temporomandibular joints often respond to local injection treatment. Symptoms responding include pain on chewing, inability fully to open the mouth, swelling and local tenderness.

The injection is made with the patient relaxed in the sitting or reclining position, with the head supported. The joint line can be felt by placing the finger in front of the tragus, and the condyle of the mandible can be felt to move on opening and closing the mouth. The injection is made with a 23-gauge needle using 1% lignocaine to anaesthetise the track. Ten milligrams of hydrocortisone or 2.5 mg of triamcinolone hexacetonide is then injected into the joint (Fig. 11.9). The upper joint space is entered by inserting the needle up to the zygomatic arch and then slipping the needle just under the arch. The lower joint space is more difficult to inject, but for best results it is important to inject both joint spaces. Withdraw the needle and insert it using a posterior–

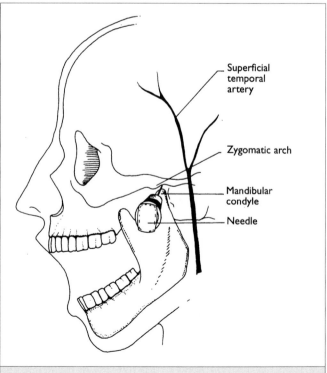

Superficial temporal artery

Zygomatic arch

Mandibular condyle

Needle

Fig. 11.9 Injection into temporomandibular joint.

inferior approach to enter the joint space at the supero-posterior aspect of the condyle.

SUMMARY OF TEMPOROMANDIBULAR EXAMINATION

- Inspection for facial asymmetry or swelling; teeth for caries and deformity.

- Inspection during movement: open mouth wide; protrude jaw forwards; move jaw laterally.
- Palpation: swelling, tenderness, lateral pterygoids.
- Resisted active movements: jaw opening, jaw closing, lateral deviation.

12

Posture and gait

Posture is the position of the body adopted when standing or sitting. Locomotion is the translation of standing posture into walking. Gait is the description of the manner of walking (or running).

POSTURE

THE EVOLUTION OF STANDING POSTURE

The length and strength of the lower limbs, the instruments of support and locomotion, are very striking and peculiar to humans. They are equal in length to the trunk and head together in normal subjects, but limb length is greater in Marfan's syndrome. The gluteus maximus, rudimentary in many animals, is the largest muscle of the human body, because of its importance in upright stance.

The *feet* are the only surface of support and are the primary agents of locomotion; they are characterised by

- longitudinal and transverse arches to allow efficient transfer of weight and stress;
- rigidity in a closed kinetic chain with strong ligamentous support to provide mechanical advantage and a rigid lever.

MECHANISMS OF CONTROL OF POSTURE

Structural locking

The locking mechanism permits standing posture of the lower limbs with little muscular activity once a static position is achieved.

The capsule of the *hip joint* is progressively twisted and shortened as the thigh extends. When full extension is reached, the surfaces are fully congruent and no further extension is possible. The *knee joint* locks in extension, block-ing further extension, and can hold a position without muscular action, provided that the weight line for the body above the knee falls in front of the centre of rotation of the joint. The joints of the *hindfoot* (subtalar and midtarsal) lock and unlock simultaneously at heel-strike and forefoot loading, thus providing an efficient rigid lever and shock absorption, respectively.

Muscular activity in posture control

During normal standing, activity is usually found in soleus and gastrocnemius, but consistent activity is usually absent in ankle dorsiflexors, quadriceps and hamstrings.

Under loads of 50–100 kg the passive structures (ligaments, etc.) appear sufficient to control joint position, but over 200 kg the muscles come progressively into play. The first line of defence, therefore, of the arches of the feet is ligamentous, while the muscles form a dynamic reserve called upon reflexly by excessive loads, including the take-off phase in walking.

Stretch reflexes

These can be regarded as a control system that can keep constant or rather nearly constant, the length of the muscle. For a system to become self-balancing, the muscle must be sensitive to the extent of the load and become quiescent when the load falls.

SENSORY FUNCTION IN POSTURE AND GAIT

Optimum control of balance, with the effects of gravity, requires continuous monitoring of body position. Control of posture and gait in humans involves the activation of pre-programmed patterns of muscle activity which are initiated and modulated by complex control pathways. These carry information from the eyes, the labyrinths and somatosensory sources, providing details of the postural effects of muscle activity. In a healthy individual these sensory inputs provide more information than is normally necessary, so that it is not critical if information from one sensory source is lost, for example by eye closure.

PHYSIOLOGICAL SENSORY IMBALANCE

This can be demonstrated in the normal subject by removing one sensory input (eye closure) and then reducing the reliability of information from other sources (attempt to balance on one foot with the head fully extended, a position in which the vestibular apparatus no longer functions optimally). This head extension vertigo (Brandt, 1981) is an example of physiological imbalance. The experience of vertigo is linked to impaired perception of a stationary environment. Although lack of one sensory channel rarely manifests as clinically significant instability in everyday life, the demands of balancing tasks in some sports do mean that such a deficit may declare itself by instability during competition. If the history suggests this, it is important to recreate the conditions in which it is encountered.

EXAMINATION

A careful check should be made of the posture adopted in the normal standing position and in sitting. Examine from in front and then standing behind the subject. Note:

- the position of the head and neck (Fig. 12.1),
- any difference in the height at which the shoulders are held (Fig. 12.1),
- the line of the thoracolumbar spine,
- the alignment of the iliac crests (Fig. 12.1),
- the position of the patellae and alignment of the knee (Fig. 12.2),
- the position of the feet (pronated or supinated) (Fig. 12.3).
- the height of the medial arch (pes cavus or planus, p. 115)

Assess whether abnormal posture is spinal (*see* Chapter 7) or related to lower limb change.

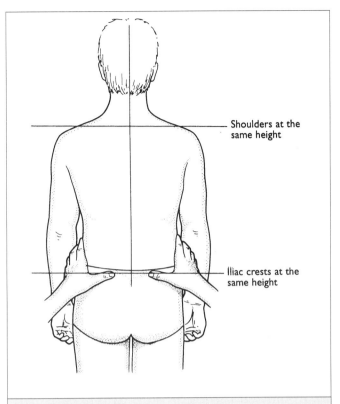

Fig. 12.1 Normal posture.

Shoulders at the same height

Iliac crests at the same height

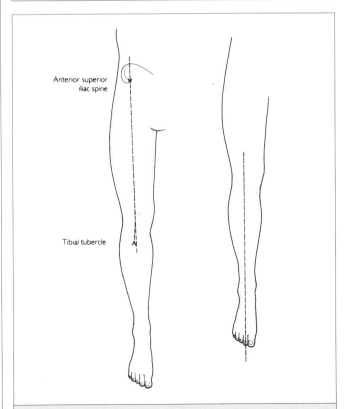

Anterior superior iliac spine

Tibial tubercle

Fig. 12.2 Normal standing posture of the lower right limb. When the foot is neutral the middle of the patella should align approximately with the second toe.

Fig. 12.3 Normal hindfoot posture (neutral subtalar joint in the prone position).

Examination for lower limb causes of abnormal posture

Leg length inequality

This can be assessed with the patient standing, by noting a tilt in a line drawn across from the posterior superior iliac spine (compare Fig. 12.1 and Fig. 12.7). Formal measurement is made by tape measure from the anterior superior iliac spine to the medial malleolus of the ankle and comparison made with the opposite side (Fig. 12.4). Discrepancy confirms *true leg length inequality*. The site of the shortening should be determined if possible by direct comparison with the opposite side (Fig. 12.5). Measurement inequality from umbilicus to medial malleoli indicates *apparent shortening*.

An inequality of about 2 cm or more tends to overload lower limb joints, because of changes in load line. In runners the effects are often amplified and smaller inequalities may become important.

Miserable malalignment syndrome

In this syndrome there is internal rotation of the tibia, the calcaneum everts and the forefoot abducts on the rearfoot as the talus adducts. The medial longitudinal arch is lowered and the foot relatively dorsiflexes, so that the centre of gravity (load line) is medial to the foot: this results in functional

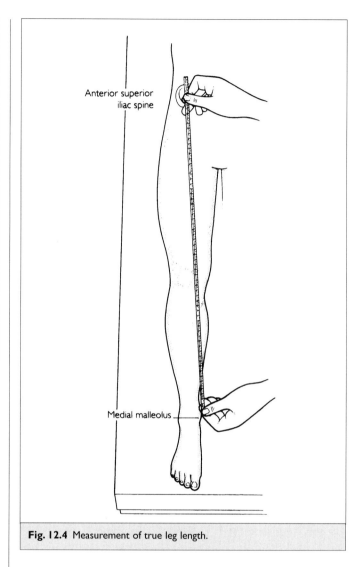

Fig. 12.4 Measurement of true leg length.

valgus at the knee with functional increased Q-angle (Fig. 12.6). Quadriceps contraction pulls the patella laterally.

This syndrome can produce, particularly in runners:

- patellofemoral pain;
- medial tibial pain (shin splints) due to overstressing of the tibialis posterior, as it attempts to counteract excessive pronation;
- stretching of the deltoid ligament and the lateral ligament of the ankle;
- medial plantar fascial stretch;
- abductovalgus deformity of the hallux.

Excessive unilateral foot pronation

Here, calcaneal valgus and functional valgus at the knee are seen (Fig. 12.7). These result in a *functionally short leg* and a postural scoliosis, correcting on sitting or lying. The right

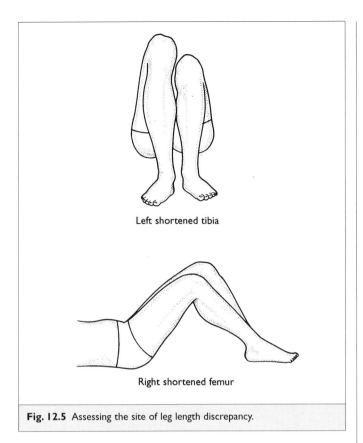

Left shortened tibia

Right shortened femur

Fig. 12.5 Assessing the site of leg length discrepancy.

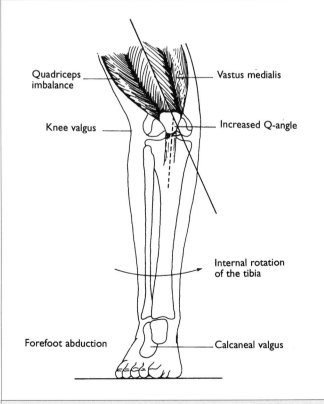

Quadriceps imbalance

Vastus medialis

Knee valgus

Increased Q-angle

Internal rotation of the tibia

Forefoot abduction

Calcaneal valgus

Fig. 12.6 Functional valgus resulting from miserable malalignment syndrome.

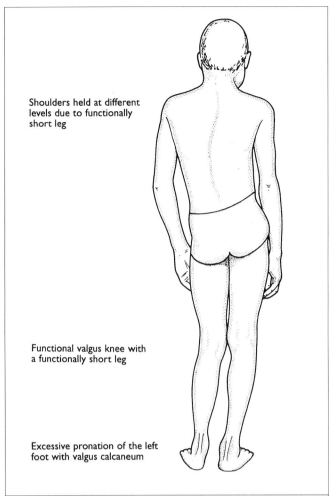

Shoulders held at different levels due to functionally short leg

Functional valgus knee with a functionally short leg

Excessive pronation of the left foot with valgus calcaneum

Fig. 12.7 Functionally short left leg with compensatory scoliosis.

scapula is lower than the left and there is compensation at the cervical region.

The load line

The *load line* in standing is *vertical* from the position of the *centre of mass*. Standing on one foot—if possible—will indicate the position of the load line in relation to lower limb joints. A load line passing to one side of a joint indicates a turning moment being applied to that joint through the body weight, resulting in potential soft-tissue strain and joint wear. Running, and particularly road-running, will frequently bring out relatively minor loading abnormalities and produce sports injuries of the overuse type. It is vital, therefore, that management involves both short-term treatment of the injury and correction of any imbalance by referral, if possible, to an experienced podiatrist with expertise in running injuries.

GAIT

Normal gait is a complete coordinated sum of the body's movement which results in forward progression of the body in the desired direction. It involves all segments of the body, in weight-bearing, in counterbalancing motion, or in maintaining correct alignment and orientation of the body parts. The integration of all these activities must be coordinated and simultaneous, since interference with a single part will result in altered function of the remaining components.

Walking is a process of extraordinary complexity, in which multiple individual motions occur at many sites simultaneously in the three planes of space. In the biomechanics of locomotion there is a long chain of interlinked mechanisms from spine to distal toe. The six major determinants of gait are:

- pelvic rotation,
- pelvic tilt,
- lateral pelvic displacement,
- knee extension and flexion,
- ankle joint dorsiflexion,
- subtalar and midtarsal joint function.

Should there be a fault in the system, since there is a large amount of 'engineering redundancy', compensation usually occurs elsewhere so that the individual's mobility is retained. However, this compensation may later cause mechanical stress because forces are being transmitted through the wrong anatomical site or may become greater than the design limits. Bone and soft tissues increase in strength in response to extra loading, but joint surfaces may be damaged by unusual loading forces.

The human race is more suited to natural surfaces with varying terrain, allowing a variety of foot plant, joint positions and muscle function, hence the use of various functional motor units. We have not evolved adaptations to hard unyielding artificial surfaces, as shown by the high injury rate in road runners. This is reflected in the rapid impact spike seen in running on hard surfaces, but not on natural surfaces, which decreases the rate of impact motion.

A brief review of the biomechanics of normal walking is essential to the understanding of abnormal walking patterns.

Gait cycle

The phases of the normal gait cycle are illustrated in Fig. 12.8 and comprise:

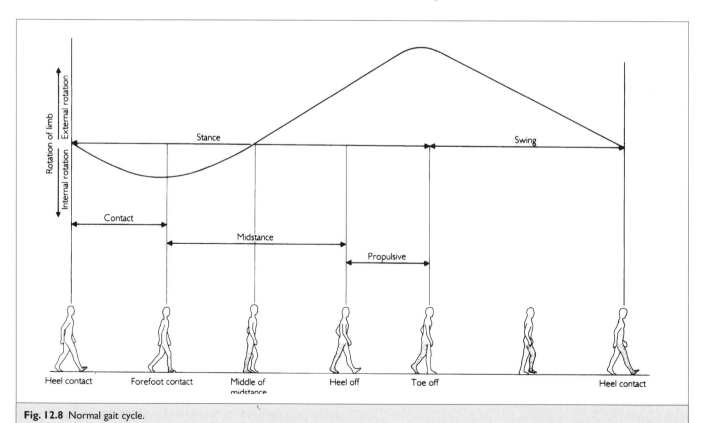

Fig. 12.8 Normal gait cycle.

- heel contact,
- forefoot contact,
- heel-off,
- toe-off.

The components of these phases (illustrated in Fig. 12.9) can be summarised as follows.

Heel contact phase/forefoot contact phase: *the tibialis anterior* dorsiflexes the ankle and inverts the foot and so prevents the sudden slap of excess plantar flexion: it also supinates the forefoot with initial lateral heel contact. The forefoot loads from lateral to medial as the tibialis anterior relaxes and the forefoot everts. There is deceleration of rearfoot pronation by *tibialis posterior* which also reduces internal rotation of the leg when the forefoot touches the ground. *Flexor digitorum longus* and *gastrocnemii* (which also maintain knee flexion) complete subtalar deceleration.

Midstance: There is deceleration of anterior momentum of the leg and knee extension (*gastrocnemii* simultaneously tense, preventing knee hyperextension). There is acceleration of subtalar, supination and tibial external rotation.

Linear acceleration of the trunk carries the femur and tibia forward over the foot, so the ankle dorsiflexes and heel lifts.

There is stabilisation of the lesser tarsus, metatarsus and rays 2, 3 and 4 and stabilisation of 1st ray metatarsus and cuneiform) and 5th metatarsus.

Propulsive phase: With heel-lift, the ankle joint plantar flexes. There is transverse stabilisation of the metatarsal heads and medial transfer of body weight. Propulsion occurs through the lesser digits acting as a rigid beam and the hallux with sesamoid sliding function.

Swing phase: Following toe-off (forefront clearance) the ankle and 1st ray dorsiflex, the forefoot supinates at metatarsus and there is rearfoot pronation at the subtalar joint. Heel contact occurs at the end of the swing phase and the next cycle starts.

EXAMINATION

It is best to assess gait with the legs and feet fully exposed. Ask the patient to walk away from you, to turn at an agreed point and then to walk back towards you.

Fig. 12.9 Phases of the gait cycle (see text for details of components of each phase).

If the gait is abnormal, it must be analysed more fully to define whether this is due to a lower limb problem or neurological disorder. Intoxication, hysteria or malingering may occasionally cause difficulty in diagnosis.

Simple causes, such as a painful corn or osteoarthritis will be confirmed by full examination of the lower limbs.

Since an altered gait due to pain will often lead to unusual stresses being placed on soft tissues, the patient will often present with this secondary pain. It is vital therefore that the clinician uncovers the original mechanical problem. Adequate evaluation of an athlete presenting with pain should ideally include a treadmill assessment of running pattern. Equally, a patient with rheumatoid arthritis needs careful assessment of walking pattern to evaluate the contribution of mechanical factors complicating either established joint deformity or altered gait due to pain. Suitable orthotics may considerably improve locomotion, but inappropriate prescription may worsen symptoms. It is the clinician's role to evaluate which patients merit referral.

Neurological patterns of gait disturbance

Neurological causes should be diagnosed on the basis of the following well-recognised abnormal patterns and confirmed by a full neurological examination.

A *narrow-based, dragging gait* is typical of *spasticity*. The patient has difficulty bending the knees, dragging the feet along as if glued to the floor. On a hard surface this can be heard as well as seen. The foot is raised from the ground by the patient tilting the pelvis and swinging the lower limb forward in an arc of circumduction, with the toes scraping along the floor. This is unilateral in the hemiplegic gait, the asymmetry making the pelvic tilt and circumduction swing of the affected leg more striking.

A *'scissor-like' gait* is seen when there is adduction and internal rotation of the hips with an equinus of the feet and flexion at the knee.

A *wide-based stamping gait* is typical of *sensory ataxia* and best seen in tabes dorsalis. The patient raises the foot suddenly and usually high, then jerks the foot forward before bringing it to the ground again with a stamp. The eyes are usually fixed to the ground to help compensate for the loss of position sense. With the eyes closed the patient will stumble or fall and often notices the problem for the first time in the dark or on stairs.

A *wide-based staggering or 'reeling' gait* is seen in *cerebellar ataxia*. The feet are wide apart and are planted irregularly, with the arms often flung out to improve balance. There may also be associated titubation, a rhythmical shaking movement of body and head. The ataxia is the same with the eyes opened or closed.

A *stooping, festinant gait* is characteristic of *Parkinson's disease*. The posture is stooped due to a flexion dystonia, and the arms do not swing, often being flexed against the body. There is a slowness in starting, but after small, shuffling steps there is a tendency to break into a tottering (festinant) run. In some patients, if suddenly pulled from behind, they begin to walk backwards and find it difficult to stop (retropulsion).

A *rapid, short-stepped gait* (*marche à petits pas*) with a tapping quality is seen in deep cerebral corticospinal lesions.

The combination of an ataxic gait and weakness, for example in *subacute combined degeneration of the cord*, may result in an increasingly irregular gait with a tendency for the knees to give way suddenly.

The involuntary movements of chorea or dystonia are usually increased on walking and unusual responses may occur when the feet are planted, for example an *avoiding response*, when the toes extend away from the floor, or the *grasping response*, when the feet appear stuck to the floor.

A *waddling gait*, like a duck, is due to the problem of maintaining truncal and pelvic posture, caused by *proximal muscle weakness*, in proximal myopathies, including polymyositis and osteomalacia, and muscular dystrophies. The body tends to be tilted backwards with increased lumbar lordosis and the body sways from side to side, due to the gluteal muscle weakness, as each step is taken. A similar gait can be seen in bilateral hip joint disease with secondary muscle weakness (*Trendelenburg gait*).

A *high-stepping gait*, with a slap of the foot in the contact phase, because ankle plantar flexion is unrestrained, is seen in weakness of tibialis anterior (foot drop).

TYPICAL GAITS OF MECHANICAL DISORDERS

Congenital dislocation

1. *Unilateral*: the child lurches to the affected side, because of poor gluteal muscles, shortening of the femoral neck and displacement of the femoral head, as well as lumbar lordosis and abnormal lateral mobility.
2. *Bilateral*: waddling gait ('duck-like' or 'sailor's' gait), inclining to each side on weight-bearing.

Coxa vara

- Waddling gait.
- Stands with leg externally rotated and slightly abducted, pelvis tilted down on the affected side.
- There is usually a slight lumbar scoliosis towards the affected side.
- Buttock atrophied, gluteal fold lower.
- Greater trochanter lower on the affected side.

Infective, inflammatory or degenerative hip disease

Gait is lurching over the involved hip in order to reduce impact on the hip (*antalgic gait*). The child with infective or inflammatory disease tends to adopt a position of hip flexion, abduction or adduction with external rotation. This produces some degree of increased lumbar lordosis.

Club foot: congenital talipes equinovarus

The gait is stumbling, due to lack of elasticity. If unilateral the deformity is usually less severe, but the leg is obviously smaller and less well-developed. Essential signs are:

- plantar flexion of the talus,
- inversion of calcaneum (and other tarsals),
- adduction of the forefoot,
- muscles poorly developed and tendons attenuated,
- plantar muscles contracted, but anterior leg muscles elongated.

Note: the inverted foot position is frequently adopted by normal young infants.

EXAMINATION OF CHILDREN

When assessing the posture of a child, examination must be performed with the child *lying, sitting and standing*. Note any abnormal movements or response to movement. Examine for hyperlaxity of joints and for muscle tone. Note, with the child standing, abnormalities in cervical, thoracic and lumbar spine.

When examining very young children, it is important to screen for developmental delay by comparing the child's achievements with the average for children of the same age. It is therefore important to know the normal *average* milestones of development. Table 12.1 gives a brief guide in terms of posture and walking.

Shortening

On finding true shortening in the child, determine the cause by examining for:

- *Shortness of femur or tibia*, by direct comparison and measurement (Fig. 12.6): this can be due to fracture or premature epiphyseal closure (consider skeletal dysplasia if bilateral).
- *Soft-tissue contractures*, with flexion deformity of hip, knee or ankle.
- *Joint disease of the hip*: congenital dislocation, slipped femoral epiphysis.
- *Knee disorders*: congenital genu valgum or varum.
- *Foot conditions*: congenital metatarsus varus, peroneal spastic foot, club foot deformity (congenital talipes equinovarus).

Table 12.1. Postural and walking development

Baby bringing head in line with the trunk when pulled from supine to sitting	16 weeks
The head can be held steady and erect	20 weeks
Bounce	28 weeks
Sit alone, leaning forward on hands	28 weeks
Stand steadily, *with* support for short periods	36 weeks
Sit steadily without any spinal kyphosis	40 weeks
Walk *without* support	12 months
Run, stiffly	18 months
Run without falling	24 months

Aspiration and injection techniques

Principles of joint aspiration and steroid injection

Injection techniques are easily learned and some knowledge of the easiest routes for each joint is of value to all doctors. Both diagnostic and therapeutic joint aspiration are often necessary in emergencies. Confidence is gained by studying diagrams, watching clinicians and finally by using the techniques.

Aspiration of synovial fluid (SF) is essential to confirm diagnosis whenever the cause of the inflamed joint could be septic arthritis, crystal synovitis or a haemarthrosis (Table 13.1). It may also be helpful in the differential diagnosis of inflammatory and non-inflammatory joint disease. Therapeutic aspiration is sometimes necessary to remove blood, pus or large effusions. Infected SF and blood should always be aspirated; infected SF is chondrolytic and leads to joint breakdown, and blood is an irritant and leads to synovitis. Infection often involves a single joint and usually there is marked inflammation with severe pain, tenderness, erythema and swelling. There may be minimal signs of inflammation in patients receiving corticosteroids or with a debilitating illness. In an infant, there may also be little systemic illness and the child may present with sudden refusal to move a limb.

Injection of substances into synovial joints is most commonly a therapeutic procedure and a variety of corticosteroid preparations are used. Its local effect in preventing recurrent effusion and pain may be dramatic. Although most peripheral joints can be treated in this way, this therapy should only be considered when one or possibly two joints are actively inflamed whilst others are controlled by drug treatment. Corticosteroid injections are often helpful in treating inflammatory synovitis, bursitis, nodules and lesions of tendons or at muscle insertions. Occasionally, radioisotopes are injected for therapeutic or diagnostic purposes and radio-opaque media for diagnosis.

Rheumatoid arthritis and osteoarthritis are the most common diseases for which aspiration and injection is helpful, but it can be given in any condition in which the pain is *believed to be the result of inflammation*. These include psoriatic arthropathy, ankylosing spondylitis with peripheral arthritis, Reiter's disease and pyrophosphate arthropathy. Injections may also be useful in osteoarthrosis in the acute inflammatory episodes that punctuate the course of the disease, but the use in this condition is more controversial.

The patients who are likely to benefit are those with warm swollen joints, with effusions and stiffness in the mornings. Those less likely to benefit are those with crepitus, instability and severe X-ray changes. The benefit of intra-articular injection is variable, but if it is effective it will produce its maximum benefit within a few days. In successful cases, the benefits may last for months, but often it is only for a few days. *The first injection is usually the most successful*. There is strong anecdotal evidence that the response in small joints is longer lasting than in larger joints.

The major contraindication to intrasynovial steroid administration is the presence of infection, and this procedure should, therefore, never be performed without a definite diagnosis and, if indicated, synovial fluid examination. Stringent aseptic precautions are required to minimise the risk of septic arthritis. Repeated injections may result in joint destruction resembling a neuropathic joint, and for this reason it is often recommended that weight-bearing should be *reduced* immediately after an injection. Complications are listed in Table 13.2.

Hollander introduced this therapy over 40 years ago (Hollander *et al.*, 1951) and since then a number of potent steroids have been developed. The purpose is to find a

Table 13.1. Indication for aspiration of a joint

Septic arthritis
Haemarthrosis
Crystal synovitis
Acute large effusion
Effusion interfering with function

Table 13.2. Complications of steroid injections

1. Skin atrophy at site of injection
2. Short-term facial flushing
3. Pain may be increased in the first day following injection. Microcrystalline steroid deposits may create a crystal synovitis
4. Temporary loss of diabetic control in 'brittle' diabetics
5. Tendon rupture if an intratendinous injection is given
6. Infection

suitable potent preparation with a prolonged effect after injection into joints. It is also important that there are a minimum of local side-effects (e.g. flare-ups, cystic degeneration of bone or bone resorption) and, as the synovial cavity has good absorbitive capacity, a minimum of systemic side-effects (Oka and Lähdesmäki, 1980; Armstrong *et al.*, 1981).

Some corticosteroid preparations are crystalline and may induce an acute crystal synovitis if injected into a joint. Long-acting preparations such as methylprednisolone acetate and triamcinolone hexacetonide may prolong the effect of intra-articular injection and are particularly useful in chronic diseases such as rheumatoid arthritis.

The indications for intra-articular and local steroids are as summarised in Table 13.3. It is the treatment of choice for enthesopathies; i.e. conditions such as tennis elbow in which the inflammatory process is localised to the junction of tendon or ligament and bone. Recurrences are not uncommon but the injection can be repeated.

PROCEDURE

The risk of iatrogenic infection is minimal when a careful aseptic or no-touch technique and disposable syringes and needles are used. Single-dose ampoules should be used whenever possible. Sterile towels and gloves and masks are unnecessary. One needs:

- 1% chlorhexidine in spirit or a weak solution of iodine, for skin preparation.
- A selection of needles and syringes.

Table 13.3. Indications for injection

INTRA-ARTICULAR
1. Relief of pain resulting from inflammatory arthritis localised to one or a few joints
2. Joint synovitis unresponsive to drugs
3. To aid the correction of deformity

LOCAL
1. The enthesopathies, e.g. tennis elbow
2. Compression neuropathies, e.g. carpal tunnel syndrome
3. Tenosynovitis
4. Epidural injection of steroid useful in acute lumbar disc prolapse with root compression

- Specimen bottles for the aspirates.
- Local anaesthetic (without adrenaline).
- Steroid for injection: hydrocortisone acetate suspension (20 mg/ml), methylprednisolone acetate (Depo-Medrone) (40 mg/ml), triamcinolone hexacetonide (Lederspan).
- Forceps for freeing needles jammed into syringes.
- Gauze, swabs and dressings.
- A crêpe bandage (if the effusion is large, this is helpful afterwards).
- Saline can be useful to distend the joint and mimic an effusion if no fluid is obtained.

General points

Careful palpation of bony margins and surfaces before skin preparation increases the likelihood of first-time success, and the site for skin puncture is easily indicated with a thumb-nail mark. In most cases the joint should be approached from its extensor aspect, as vulnerable neurovascular structures usually lie on the flexor aspect. Chlorhexidine in spirit or a weak iodine solution should be applied generously for skin preparation. Towels can be used for prolonged procedures such as arthrography.

To minimise discomfort during or after a corticosteroid injection it often helps to give a 1 or 2% solution of lignocaine without adrenaline first, infiltrating skin and underlying tissues down to and including the pain-sensitive joint capsule. A refrigerant spray can also be used to numb the skin. With skill and practice, rapid insertion of the needle into the joint is possible, in which case local anaesthetic can be mixed with the corticosteroid or may not be required. In some instances local anaesthetic can provide diagnostic information and may also reduce post-injection pain.

The patient

The patient should be relaxed. Tense muscles can make injection impossible, and in most instances it is best if the patient is lying supine with the head comfortably supported on pillows. This also will make it easy to treat a vasovagal attack. Having a nurse present also helps to reassure the patient and is helpful in positioning the limb correctly.

How often to inject

A good general guide is not to inject the same joint more frequently than every 4 months without considering a change in other therapy (e.g. second-line drugs in rheumatoid arthritis). The possible damage caused by frequent injection is thought to be slight, and unsuppressed inflammation is probably more damaging than the possible adverse effects of a local corticosteroid.

Choosing a needle

A 21-gauge (green) needle is sufficient for most aspirations, but a 19-gauge (white) needle may be needed for very large effusions or for fibrinous synovial fluid. A 23-gauge (blue) needle is used for aspiration of the interphalangeal joints and for most injections without aspiration.

Synovial fluid analysis

If there is the possibility of infection, the synovial fluid should be sent for Gram stain, total and differential white blood cell count, bacterial culture and polarised light microscopy for crystals (discussed in Chapter 14).

Precautions

Corticosteroid should not be injected if septic arthritis is a possibility, or if there is sepsis elsewhere. Always attempt aspiration of fluid and, if in doubt about infection, do not inject but wait for the result of microscopy and culture. Aspiration of a joint containing a prosthesis should only be done with the knowledge and advice of an orthopaedic surgeon.

When injecting soft-tissue lesions the needle should be jammed well onto the syringe before injecting, as considerable force may be needed.

The patient should be advised that post injection pain may occur that may require analgesia.

The patient should be advised against unreasonable use of the joint for 24 hours after injection. This will depend both on the nature of the lesion and on the kind of work the patient does. To minimise time off work, injections can be done just prior to the weekend. Exercise should be avoided during this period.

Dosage

For large joints (e.g. the knee) the usual dose of corticosteroid is 50 mg of hydrocortisone acetate, or 40 mg of methylprednisolone or 20 mg of triamcinolone hexacetonide. For small joints half of these doses will be needed. It is usual to use longer acting steroids for joint injections and hydrocortisone for soft-tissue injections. Longer acting steroids may lead to fat atrophy if used for soft-tissue lesions.

In a large joint, be sure to use an adequate amount of fluid because, particularly in the knee, an injection of corticosteroid alone tends to remain in one place unless diluted.

Follow-up and advice

All patients given an injection should be seen again to make sure that symptoms have improved and that no complications have occurred. Advice should include the following:

- The joint may be painful for up to 24 hours after the injection.
- It may take several days for benefit to occur following the injection.
- The injected joint should be rested if possible for 24–48 hours.
- No sport should be contemplated for at least 5 days.
- Supportive splints, such as a forearm band for tennis elbow, may prevent a recurrence of the injury.

Failure to respond

1. The injection may not have penetrated the joint. When training, one can put a small amount of contrast medium in the syringe and X-ray afterwards to check.
2. The main cause of the joint pain was not inflammatory arthritis, but secondary osteoarthritis.

Individual joints

Procedures for individual joints are discussed at the end of each chapter in the previous section.

Examination of synovial fluid

Examination of synovial or bursal fluid is particularly important in the diagnosis of two treatable conditions, acute sepsis and crystal-associated disease. Synovial fluid (SF) findings may also be of diagnostic significance in a few rare diseases (e.g. amyloid), but for most other conditions SF abnormalities, while often supporting the presumed diagnosis, are non-specific.

For clinical purposes, SF examinations to consider include:

- macroscopic appearance (colour, clarity, viscosity),
- cell count and differential,
- light microscopy,
- polarised microscopy (for crystal identification),
- Gram stain and culture,
- special tests in limited situations.

GENERAL ASPECTS OF SF COLLECTION AND STORAGE

Although the options for SF analysis are to some extent determined by the *volume* aspirated, even very small amounts may suffice to make a diagnosis. Even if an apparently '*dry tap*' is obtained at aspiration:

- the contents of the needle should still be expelled onto a slide and examined for crystals (unsuspected minute SF drops are often present), or
- if sepsis is strongly suspected, consider injecting the joint with sterile saline and sending the aspirated washings for culture.

For small amounts of SF the usual priorities are a couple of drops onto an alcohol-cleaned, dry microscope slide, the rest being retained for culture. If a larger amount is obtained, it is usual to divide the sample into two sterile plain containers, one for culture and one for crystal identification (anticoagulants added are crystalline and confound crystal analysis). With larger volumes, additional aliquots to consider may include:

- 4 ml into an EDTA tube (e.g. for total and differential leucocyte counts by Coulter counter, or for estimation of complement breakdown products), and
- direct inoculation into blood-culture bottles (for both aerobic and anaerobic organisms).

The volume of aspirated SF can itself be a measure of arthritis severity. Low volumes, however, do not necessarily negate an important intra-articular process: SF may be loculated and fibrin, rice bodies and other debris may hinder 'aspiration to dryness'.

It is always preferable to examine SF as fresh as possible. Problems that arise if analysis is delayed include:

- a decrease in cell count (due to disruption),
- partial dissolution and decrease in number of readily detectable crystals (calcium pyrophosphate > urate), and
- appearance of post-aspiration artefactual crystals.

Storage at 4°C will retard but not prevent such changes and SF ideally should be examined within 4 hours of aspiration.

MACROSCOPIC APPEARANCE: COLOUR, CLARITY AND VISCOSITY

Normal SF is colourless or pale yellow: it contains few cells (< 50/μl: mainly mononuclear) and little debris, and therefore appears clear. Its hyaluronic acid content and degree of polymerisation impart high viscosity which can be crudely assessed by allowing SF to drop from the needle tip (normal and 'non-inflammatory' SF both form a 'string' up to 2–5 cm long before separating). Owing to the absence of fibrinogen and clotting factors (particularly prothrombin and factors V and VII), normal SF does not clot.

In general, *'non-inflammatory'* SF appears similar to normal SF, whilst *'inflammatory'* SF shows a tendency to:

- decreased viscosity (forming a short string and dropping more like water),
- increased turbidity (due to increased cells, fibrin strands, debris, Plate 1 (reproduced courtesy of Dieppe *et al.*, 1986),
- deepening colour (yellow/orange/green),
- spontaneous clot formation.

Greatly increased viscosity suggests hypothyroidism (or recent steroid injection into that joint).

Blood staining is very common and usually caused by the trauma of the aspiration. If it is uniform, however, causes of true haemarthrosis need to be considered (Table 14.1). A lipid layer overlying a haemarthrosis suggests intra-articular fracture. Uniformly *milky* white SF may result from plentiful cholesterol or urate crystals.

Rice bodies are small, glistening, white objects (mainly fibrin and collagen) which represent sloughed microinfarcted synovial villi. They are a non-specific finding in severe synovitis (e.g. rheumatoid and tuberculous arthritis). Much smaller, black particles are a rare finding in SF from ochronotic joints (*ground-pepper* sign).

CELL COUNT AND DIFFERENTIAL

Cells can be counted using a Coulter counter or cell counting chamber and microscope (Wright's stain, or haematoxylin and eosin are suitable for differential counts). Transport in an EDTA tube often facilitates cell counting.

In general, the total count and proportion of polymorphs increase with severity of inflammation, the cell count being one of the features used to classify SF as 'non-inflammatory' (200–2000 cells/µl) or 'inflammatory' (>2000 cells/µl). The differential is more useful than the total cell count, although both lack specificity and show considerable overlap between conditions. Nevertheless, in general:

Table 14.1. Principal causes of haemarthrosis

COMMON
Trauma
Severe inflammatory or destructive arthropathy
  (e.g. pyrophosphate arthropathy, rheumatoid arthritis, sepsis)

UNCOMMON
Bleeding disorder
  (e.g. haemophilia, anticoagulant therapy, scurvy)
Pigmented villonodular synovitis
Abnormal vessels
  (e.g. haemangioma)

- a differential count of *> 90% polymorphs* is likely to reflect acute crystal synovitis, acute sepsis or active rheumatoid arthritis;
- a differential count of *< 50% polymorphs* is likely to reflect osteoarthritis or mechanical derangement;
- a *marked monocytosis* suggests viral infection (particularly hepatitis B and rubella) or serum sickness.

CONVENTIONAL LIGHT MICROSCOPY

Occasionally, abnormal cells may be identified, including:

- *polymorphs ('ragocytes')* with multiple cytoplasmic inclusions, most commonly seen in but not specific to rheumatoid arthritis, and
- *macrophages (Reiter's cells)* containing ingested polymorphs, a non-specific finding first noted in acute Reiter's syndrome.

Apart from cells, frequent findings include *cartilage fragments* (Plate 2), *fibrin clots*, and unidentifiable *debris*. *Lipid droplets* (which stain red using oil red O) are occasionally seen in severe synovitis (e.g. rheumatoid), and may be particularly abundant in synovial or bursal fluid of patients with pancreatic arthropathy.

POLARISED MICROSCOPY

This is the usual method for routine identification of crystalline particles, although more definitive methods are required if confident identification is required (particularly for non-urate crystals). A good quality, dedicated microscope with a rotating stage will greatly facilitate crystal identification, particularly of smaller, less brightly birefringent particles.

A few drops of fresh unspun SF are usually examined, although centrifugation and examination of the deposit increases positive identification (electron microscopy of apparently negative deposits increases positive identification even further). If examination of the slide is going to be delayed, the edges of the cover slip should be sealed (using clear nail-varnish or a commercial sealant) to prevent dehydration and artefactual changes. It is very important to use a clean slide and cover slip, and to maintain the microscope as dust-free as possible. There is a marked variation in the 'cleanliness' of slides from different manufacturers, but clean untampered slides are probably ideal. If slides require cleaning, birefringent lens tissue fibres may be introduced; a reasonable compromise is to use alcohol- or acetone-cleaned slides dried in non-turbulent air.

To search for birefringent material it is easiest to scan using a low-power lens with the polarising lenses crossed (i.e. a black background). Once birefringent material is identified, the compensator and a higher power lens (×400) are used for detailed observation: oil immersion lenses are helpful for small particles. Crystals often associate with fibrin strands and cellular debris, and such areas are worthy of special scrutiny. Crystals tend to have clearly defined edges with straight sides, in contrast to the less well-defined, indistinct forms of many artefacts. Extracellular crystals are often more easily seen, but intracellular crystals should also be sought.

Crystal identification is principally on the basis of:

- size,
- morphology,
- sign of birefringence (positive or negative, according to the convention of the optics of the microscope),
- extinction angle (the angle by which the stage must be rotated for the crystal to alter from maximum to no birefringence).

Monosodium urate monohydrate (MSUM) crystals

These, the most important crystals to identify, are usually needle-shaped (acicular), ranging from 2 to 25 µm in length, and exhibiting strong (negative) birefringence and an extinction angle of 45°. Typical MSUM crystals are easy to identify with confidence (Plates 3 and 4): if any doubt exists uricase digestion of crystals is confirmatory. In synovial and bursal fluids, MSUM crystals are usually numerous and separate (either intra- or extracellular), but aggregated clumps and sheets of crystals are more typical of slides made from tophus aspirates/discharge (Plate 5).

Calcium pyrophosphate dihydrate (CPPD) crystals

These crystals are variable short, thick, usually rhomboid rods (Plates 6 and 7), 2–10 µm long, showing weak (positive) birefringence and a low extinction angle (c. 15°). With small or cuboid crystals it may be difficult to identify the long axis, and the sign of birefringence may thus appear variable or difficult to determine. Usually, CPPD crystals are present in small numbers, mainly extra- rather than intracellular, and

are easily missed. They may demonstrate 'twinning' (appearing as two conjoined crystals) and 'notches' (a chip out of one corner), and they frequently occur enmeshed in fibrin clumps and strands.

Cholesterol crystals

These are large, flat rhombic plates, 5–50 µm diameter, often with a 'folded over' corner, showing strong (mixed positive/negative) birefringence (Plate 8).

Other crystals and artefacts

Several depot *corticosteroids* are crystalline and may remain detectable in SF for several weeks following injection (Plate 9). They are variable in shape and size (usually small rods *c.* 1–8 µm), show no regular geometric form and display weak (positive or negative) birefringence. They may occur within or outside cells.

'Maltese crosses' (Plate 10) are distinctive, brightly birefringent particles that are produced by a variety of compounds (e.g. talc powder from rubber gloves, lipid, calcium oxalate, lithium heparin, dust). *Oxalate* and *lithium heparin* may also appear more rod-like and show positive birefringence. *Brushite* may rarely be seen as large, positively birefringent crystals growing as stars from a central nidus; they most commonly represent post-aspiration artefact. Fibrin strands, intracytoplasmic inclusions and hairs may all produce birefringence but lack the geometric form of arthropathy-associated crystals.

GRAM STAIN AND CULTURE

Dried smears prepared from a few drops of SF are readily stainable by Gram stain and may quickly confirm the presence of organisms (N.B.: a negative result does not exclude sepsis). The Ziehl–Neelsen stain can also be used, although identification of mycobacteria in SF is uncommon and culture and synovial biopsy are usually required for identification.

For culture of most common organisms a fresh SF sample in a sterile plain tube, speedily delivered to the microbiology department, is usually adequate. Inoculation of part of the sample into blood-culture bottles at the time of aspiration may increase the likelihood of ready identification. For suspected fastidious organisms, such as gonococcus, it may be necessary to consider transport in appropriate culture medium, or, preferably, the fluid can be plated immediately on chocolate agar or Thayer–Martin medium and the culture then continued in the laboratory under CO_2. For suspected fungal infections the fluid should be transported in a plain tube and processed for culture on Sabouraud's dextrose agar. Lowenstein's medium is used for mycobacteria. Wherever possible, particularly for potentially unusual organisms, early discussion with the microbiologist (before aspiration) is advised.

SPECIAL TESTS IN LIMITED SITUATIONS

Amyloid deposits in a spun SF deposit can be stained with Congo red, showing up as fibrillar or amorphous material with apple-green birefringence. More definitive confirmation requires examination using electron microscopy.

Apatite particles are too small to be seen by light microscopy, but aggregates can be visualised by staining with the non-specific calcium stain alizarin red S (Plate 11). At acidic pH (4.5) this stain shows better specificity for apatite than other calcium-containing crystals. Such stained aggregates are a common non-specific SF finding, but in apatite-associated destructive arthropathy they are present in large amounts.

Glucose estimation for SF placed immediately into a fluoride tube can be compared with a simultaneous serum sample (preferably fasting since equilibration between blood and SF is slow). In the presence of inflammation (e.g. rheumatoid arthritis) SF glucose falls, but very low levels (<25%) are highly suggestive of infection. Such simple estimation may be of help in some cases of chronic monoarthritis.

Most other SF investigations (e.g. complement breakdown products, autoantibodies, lactic acid, pH, cartilage matrix components) are primarily for research use and have little diagnostic significance or benefit in routine analysis.

Recommended further reading

Armstrong RD, English J, Gibson T, Chakraborty J and Marks V (1981). Serum methylprednisolone levels following intra-articular injection of methylprednisolone acetate. *Ann Rheum Dis* **40**: 571–574.

Brandt T (1981). Sensory function and posture. In: *Posture and Gait Development: Adaptation and Modulation* (Amblar B, Berthoz A and Clarac F, eds), pp. 127–136. Amsterdam: Elsevier Science Publishers.

Cyriax J (1982). Diagnosis of soft tissue lesions. *Textbook of Orthopaedic Medicine*, Vol 1, 8th edn. London: Baillière Tindall.

Department of Health and Social Security (1986). *Morbidity Statistics from General Practice. Third National Study 1981–1982*. London: HMSO.

Dieppe PA, Bacon PA, Bamji AN and Watt I (1986). *Atlas of Clinical Rheumatology*. London: Gower Medical Publishing.

Doherty M, Doherty J (1992). *Clinical Examination in Rheumatology*. London: Wolfe.

Doherty M, Dacre J, Dieppe P, Snaith M. The 'GALS' locomotor screen. *Ann Rheum Dis* 1992; **51**: 1165–1169.

Hollander JL, Brown EM, Jessar RA and Brown CY (1951). Hydrocortisone and cortisone injected into arthritic joints. *JAMA* **147**: 1629.

Hoppenfeld S (1976). *Physical Examination of the Spine and Extremities*. New York: Appleton-Century-Crofts.

Kelsey JL (1982). *Epidemiology of Musculoskeletal Disorders*, p. 194. New York: Oxford University Press.

Little H (1986). *Rheumatological Physical Examination*. London: Grune and Stratton.

Magee D (1992). *Orthopaedic Physical Assessment*, 2nd edn. Philadelphia: WB Saunders.

Oka M and Lähdesmäki K (1962). Systemic effects of large doses of hydrocortisone acetate and prednisolone acetate administered intra-articularly to patients with rheumatoid arthritis. *Acta Rheum* **8**: 192.

Owen D (1989). Aspiration and injection of joints. In: *Textbook of Rheumatology* (Kelly WN, Harris ED, Ruddy S and Sledge CB, eds), 3rd edn, Chapter 37. Philadelphia: WB Saunders.

Polley H and Hunder G (1987) *Rheumatologic Interviewing and Physical Examination of the Joints*, 2nd edn. Philadelphia: WB Saunders.

Tubiana R (1984). *Examination of the Hand and Upper Limb*. Philadelphia: WB Saunders.

Wynne-Davies R, Hall CM and Apley AG (1985). *Atlas of Skeletal Dysplasias*. London: Churchill Livingstone.

Colour plates

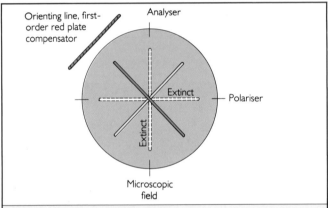

Plate 1 Macroscopic variation in synovial fluid (SF) colour, turbidity and viscosity: (1) normal, (2) 'inflammatory SF', (3) haemarthrosis, (4) milky SF (cholesterol).

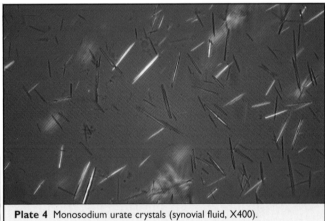

Plate 2 Cartilage fragments in synovial fluid.

Plate 3 Diagrammatic representation of a monosodium urate mono-hydrate crystal viewed down a polarising microscope.

Plate 4 Monosodium urate crystals (synovial fluid, X400).

Plate 5 Tophus aspirate (X400) showing sheets of monosodium urate monohydrate crystals.

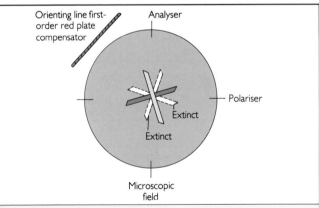

Plate 6 Diagrammatic representation of a calcium pyrophosphate dihydrate crystal viewed down a polarising microscope.

Plate 7 Calcium pyrophosphate dihydrate crystals (synovial fluid, X400).

Plate 8 Cholesterol crystals (synovial fluid, X400).

Plate 9 Triamcinolone hexacetonide crystals (synovial fluid X400) apparent 1 week after injection.

Plate 10 'Maltese crosses' due to lipid.

Plate 11 Apatite aggregates stained with alizarin red S.

Index

Numbers in *italic* refer to illustrations
and tables.

Achilles tendon, 114
  bursitis, injection, 126
  palpation, 120, 121
  ruptured, *121*
  tendinitis, 116
    injection 126
Achondroplasia, 96
Acromioclavicular joint, *31,*
  35
  assessing stability, 40
  injection, 50
  nerve supply, 35
  pain, 37, 38, 45–46
  swelling, 40
  testing, 46
Activities of daily living (ADL),
  12
Adactyly, 115
Adductor tendinitis, *89,* 92
Adhesive capsulitis, 36, 38
Adson's manoeuvre, 79
Adventitious bursae, 4
Age, shoulder pain, 36–37
American Rheumatism Association
  joint count, 24
Amyloid depostis, synovial fluid, 153
Ankle joint
  anatomy, 112–113
    ligaments, *113*
    tendons and bursae, 114, *115*
  aspiration and injection, 125, *126*
  examination
    palpation, 118-119

range of movement, 121–122
  tests of stability, 122, 123, *124*
Ankylosing spondylitis
  outcome measures, clinical
    trials, 27
  radiological scoring, 25
Anserine bursa, 104
Antalgic gait, 17–18, 90, 143
Anterior cruciate ligament, 98
Anterior drawer test
  anterior cruciate ligament, 107
  anterior talofibular ligament, 122,
    123
'Anvil' test, 92
Apatite particles, synovial fluid, 153
  plate 11
Apprehension test, anterior stability,
  glenohumeral joint, 47
Arm dominance, 37
Arthritis Impact Measurement Scales
  (AIMS), 26
Arthrocentesis, knee joint, 108–111
Arthrogaphy
  shoulder joint, 48
  temporomandibular joint, 134
Arthroscopy
  shoulder joint, 48
  temporomandibular joint, 134
Articular indices, 24
Aspiration *see* Synovial fluid:
  aspiration
Ataxia, 142
Atlanto-axial joint, 76
Atlanto-occipital joint, 76
Atlas, 73, *74*
Attitude of patient, 7, 8

Axillary nerve, 34
  entrapment, 38
Axis, 73, *74*

Baker's cyst, 104
Balloon sign, 9, *10, 103*
Barber's chair sign, 79
Biceps, 52, *53*
Biceps femoris, 98
Biceps tendon, long head, *33*
  ruptured, 39
Bicipital bursa, 104
Bicipital tendinitis, 44
  injection, 50
Birefringent material, synovial
  fluid, 152
Bony pain, 6, 7
Boutonnière deformity, *65,* 66
Brachial artery occlusion, 69
Brachial plexus lesions, 68
Brachialis, 52, *53*
Brachioradialis, 52, *53*
Brachydactyly, 115
Brushite crystals, synovial fluid, 152
Bulge sign, 9, *10*
Bulge test, 102, *103*
Bunnell's contracture, *69*
Bunnell's test, 67
Bursae, 4
  elbow joint, 53, 54
  foot and ankle, 114–*115*
  hip joint, 88, 89, 91, 92
  knee joint, 102, 103, 104
    injection, 109
  shoulder joint, 33, *34,* 36

C-reactive protein (CRP), 26
Calcium pyrophosphate dihydrate
    (CPPD)
        crystals, 152, plates 6, 7
Capsule, joint, 4
    swelling, 9
Carpal tunnel syndrome, 54
Carpetlayer's knee, 102
Carrying angle, 51
Cartilage fragments, 151, plate 2
Cauda equina, 74
    syndrome, 84
Causalgia, 62
Cell count, synovial fluid, 151
Centres of ossification, 86
Cerebellar ataxia, 142
Cervial spine
    anatomy, 72, 73, 74
    examination, 20, 47, 76–79
        observation, 76, 77, 78
        palpation, 77, 78
        range of movement, 76, 78–79
    myelopathy, 79
    spondylosis, 37
Children, posture and gait
    examination, 143
Cholesterol crystals 152, plate 8
Cinema sign, 100
Claw toe deformity, 117
Clicking, temporomandibular
    joint, 130–131
Clinical trials, disease
    measurements, 26–27
Close-packe position, 8
Clubbing, 62, 70
Clubfoot, 115, 117, 143
Coccyx, 72, 84
Collateral ligament stability, elbow
    joint, 58
Computerised tomography (CT)
    shoulder joint, 48
    temporomandibular joint, 134
Condylar growth abnormalities, 130
Congenital dislocation of hip, 86, 90
    gait disturbance, 142
Congenital skeletal abnormalities, and
    development, 3

Conjunctivitis, 14
Connective tissue disease,
    features, 64
Conversion phenomena, 62
Coracoacromial ligament, 33, 34
Corticosteroids see Steroid injection
Cosoclavicular test, 46
Coxa vera deformity of hip, 86, 143
Cracking noises, 12
Crepitus, 12
    elbow joint, 57
    shoulder joint, 38, 40
Cricoid cartilage, 76, 77
Crystals, synovial fluid, 152
Cubital fossa, 55
Cubital tunnel syndrome, 58
Culture, synovial fluid, 152–153

De Quervain's tenosynovitis, 54, 66
    Finkelstein's test, 11, 12, 66
'Dead-arm syndrome', 46
Deep bursae, 4
    deep infrapatellar bursa, 104
        injection, 109, 110
Deformity, 7, 8
Deltoid ligament insufficiency, 123
Deltoid wasting, 39
Depression, 7
Dermatomes
    around elbow, 54
    around shoulder, 37
    leg, 89
    sites of pain, 6
    spinal distribution, 75, 76
Dermatomyotosis, 64
Diabetes
    adhesive capsulitis, 36
    diabetic amyotrophy, 101
Diagnostic aspiration, 147
Diarthroses see Synovial joints
Disability, 7, 23
Discs, 4, 73
    degenerative disease, 80
    prolapse, 71
Disease assessment
    indices, disease activity, 23–25
    measurement in clinical

practice, 27
measurement of damage, 25
measurements in clinical
    trials, 26–27
outcome measures, 25–26
severity criteria, 25
Distal tibiofibular joint, 112
Dosage, steroid injections, 149
Doyle index, 24
Dressing difficulties, 16, 17
Dupuytren's contracture, 63

Elbow flexion test, 58
Elbow joint, 51–60
    aspiration and injection, 59–60
    examination, 54–59
        additional tests, 57–59
        inspection, 54, 55–56
        palpation, 56–57
    functional anatomy, 51–53
    pain, 53–54
Electromyography,
    temporomandibular joint, 134
Embroyology, 3
Emotional state, pain severity, 6
Enthesis, 4
Enthesitis, 92
Epicondylitis, 53, 54
    injection, 59–60
    testing for, 57
Epiphyseal growth deformities,
    knee, 96, 101
Episcleritis, 14
Erb's palsy, 35
    'waiter's arm' deformity, 68
Erythema, 8–9
    palmar, 14
Erythrocyte sedimentation rate
    (ESR), 26
Examination, general aspects
    minimum examination, 16–2
        lying on couch, 21–22
        standing, 18–21
        walking, 17–18
    principles of, 4–15
        assimilation of findings, 14–15
        signs, 7–13

special aspects, 13–14
symptoms, 5–7
terminology, 5
screening history, 16
Eye changes, 14
Facial asymmetry, 78
Fatigue, measurement, 24
Femoral stretch test, 83, *84*
Festinant gait, 142
Fibrin clots, 151
Fibrocartilage pads, 4
Fibromyalgia syndrome, 7, 13, 71
  outcome measures, clinical
    trials, 27
  skinfold rolling, *18*, 19
  tender sites, *13*
Finger
  adduction, assessing, *66, 67*
  clubbing, *62, 70*
  deformities, rheumatoid
    arthritis, *65*
Finkelstein's test, *11, 12*, 66
Flat foot, 115, 116–117, *119*
Flexion deformity, knee joint, 101, 106
Fluid swelling, 9, *10*
Foot, 136
  anatomy, 112, 113
    arch of foot, 113–114
    innervation, 115–116
    nerve roots, peripheral nerves
      and
        muscles involvement in
          movement, *124*
    tendons and bursae, 114–*115*
  development, 115
  examination
    excessive unilateral foot
      pronation, 138, 139
    inspection, 116–118
    muscle testing, 124–125
    palpation, 119–121
    range of movements, 122, 123,
      124
  gait problems, 17, 18
  symptoms, 115–116
Foraminal compression test, 79
Forearm supination and

pronation, 55, *56*
Forefoot problem, gait
  disturbance, 18
Fuchs index, 24

Gait, 140–143
  disturbances, 17–18, 90
    mechanical disorders, 142–143
    neurological patterns, 142
  examination, 17, 141, 142
    children, 143
  gait cycle, 17, 140–141
Gamekeeper's knee, 104
Genu recurvatum, 101
Genu valgum, 96, 101
Genu varum, 96, 101
Glenohumeral joint
  anatomy, *31*
    functional anatomy, 35
    joint capsule, 32
  assessing stability, 40, 46–47
  effusion, signs, 9
  injection, 50
  pain, 37, 38, 45
  range of movement, 41, 42, *44*
  synovitis, attitude of patient, 7
Global assessments, 25
Glucose estimation, synovial
  fluid, 153
Gluteal tendinitis, *89*
Golfer's elbow *see* Medial
  epicondylitis
Gout, in hands, 64, *65*
Gram stain, synovial fluid, 152

Haemarthrosis
  causes, *151*
  knee joint, 100
Hallux rigidus, 118
Hallux valgus, 117, *118*
Hammer toe deformity, 117
Hamstring tightness, 106
Handicap, 7, 12, 23
Hands
  examination, 20, *21*, 62–69
    acutely traumatised hand, 70
    blood supply, 69

bones and joints, 63–66
  nerves, 67, 68–69
  normal range of movement, *64*
  skin, 63
  in systemic disease, 70
  tendons and muscles, 66–67
functional anatomy, 61
pain paterns, 61–62
Health Assessment Questionnaire
  (HAQ), 26
High-stepping gait, 142
Hindfoot problem, gait
  disturbance, 17
Hip joint, 86–95
  anatomy, 87–88
    landmarks, pelvis and femur, *90*
  aspiration and injection, 95
  development, 86
    abnormalities, 86–87
  examination, 19, 21, 22, 89–94
    gait distrubance, 17, 143
    inspection, 89–91
    muscle testing, 94
    palpation, 91–92
    range of movement, 92–94, 136
  symptoms, 88–89
'Homunculus', recording locomotor
  signs, *13*
Horner's syndrome, 79
Housemaid's knee, 102
Humeroradial joint, 52
Humeroulnar ('trochlea') joint, 51
Humerus supracondylar process
  syndrome, 59
Hyaline cartilage, 4
Hyalurionic acid cysts, 65
Hydrocortisone acetate, dosage, 149
Hyoid bone, 76, 77
Hyperextension deformities,
  toes, 117, *118*
Hypermobility, generalised, 12–13,
  101
  Carter and Wilson score, *13*
Hypertrophic osteodystrophy, 62, 64
Hypochondroplasia, 96
Hypodactyly, 115
Hysterical/psychogenic gaits, 18

Idiopathic scoliosis, 80
Iliopectinal bursa, 88
    bursitis, 91, 92
Iliotibial band, 88
    contraction, 86–87
        Ober test, 93, 94
    syndrome, injection, 111
Impairment, 23
Infection, 147
Inflammation, 147
    characteristic findings, *11*
        erythema, 8–*9*
        pain, 62, 71
        warmth, 9
    synovial fluid appearance, 151
Infraspinatus muscle, 32, 33
    wasting, 39
Interphalangeal joints
    foot, 113
    hand, 61, 66
    synovitis, 9
Intertarsal joints, palpation, 119
Iritis, *14*
Ischaemia, in hand, 69
Ischiogluteal bursa, 88
    bursitis, 89
        injection 95

Jaw *see* Temporomandibular joint
Joints
    assessment of involvement, 24
    damage, signs, *11*
    development and structure, 3–4
    function, 12–13
    normal, 16–17
    pain *see* Pain
    range of movement, 10–12
    red, 8
    stability, 12
    swelling, 9–*10*
    tenderness, 10
Juvenile chronic arthritis, hands, *65*

Klumpke's deformity, 68
Knee joint, 8, 96–111
    aspiration and injection, 108–111
        approaches, 108–109

corticosteroid injection, 109
        soft-tissue injection around
            knee, 109–111
        tendinitis, 110, 111
    development, 96
    examination, 21, *22*, 101–107
        effusion, 9, 102
        gait disturbance, 17
        genu varum, valgum and
            recurvatum, 101
        muscle wasting, 101, 102
        range of movement, 105–106,
            136
Knee joint (*Cont.*)
        stability, 106–107
        tenderness, 104
    functional anatomy
        extensor mechanism, 98
        fibrous capsule, 97
        innervation and blood
            supply, 99
        intra-articular ligaments, 97–98
        menisci, 96, 97
        stability, 98–99
        surface anatomy, *99*
    history of injury, 100–101
    pain, 88, 99–100
    see also Tibiofibular joint
Kyphosis, 80, *81*

Laboratory assessment, disease
    activity, 26
Lachman's test, 106
Lateral epicondylitis, 53–54
    injection, 59–60
    testing for, 57
Leg-length discrepancy, 91, 138, *139*
    children, 143
Lhermitte's sign, 79
Ligamentous snaps, 12
Ligaments, 4
Limbs, embryological development, 3
Limping, 88
Lipid droplets, 151
Lithium heparin, in synovial
    fluid, 152
Load line, 139

Local anaesthesia, joint injection, 148
Locked
    jaw, 131
    knee, 99, 101, 106
Loose body locking, knee, 99, 101
Loose-packe position, 8
Low back problems, gait
    disturbance, 17
Lumbar spine
    anatomy, 72, 73, 74
    examination, 81–84
        malingering, tests
            suggesting, 83–84
        observation, 81
        range of movement, 82–83
        testing, 19
    lordosis, 72, *73*, *81*, 90, 91
    scoliosis, 80

McGill Pain Questionnaire, 24
McMurray's test, 106
Macrophages, 151
Malingering, tests suggesting, 83–84
Mallet finger, *65*
Mallet toe, 117
'Maltese crosses', synovial fluid, 152,
    plate 10
Manibular
    growth, developmental
        abnormalities, 130
    movement, limitation, 131
Marche à petits pas, 142
Marfan's syndrome, 63, 96, 136
Masseter muscles, palpation, 131, 132
Medial epicondylitis, 53, 54
    injection, 60
    testing for, 57
Median nerve lesions, features, 59,
    68, 69
Menisci, 4
    knee joint, 96, 97
        cysts, 102
        lateral tear, 101
        medial tear, 100–101
    temporomandibular joint, 128
        displacement, 129
Meralgia paraesthetica, *89*, 92

injection site, 95
Mesenchymal tissues, 3
Metacarpal squeeze, *21*, 64
Metacarpophalangeal (MCP)
  joints, 61
  deformities, *65*, 66
  range of movement, 64
Metatarsal squeeze, *22*
Metatarsophalangeal (MTP) joints
  anatomy, 113
  aspiration and injection of first, 126
  examination
    palpation, 119–120
    range of movement, 122, *123*, 125
  hallus valgus, 117, *118*
  hammer toe deformity, 117
  subluxation, 117, 120
Metatarsus primus varus, 115
Methylprednisolone acetate, 148
  dosage, 149
Midfoot problem, gait disturbance, 18
Midtarsal joint, 113, 136
  aspiration and injection, 126
  testing, 122, *123*
Miserable malalignment
  syndrome, 138, *139*
Monosodium urate monohydrate
  (MSUM)
  crystals, 152, plates 2, 3, 4
Morquio's syndrome, 96
Morton's neuroma, 115, 120
  injection, 127
Mouth
  examining, 133
  span, normal, 132
Movement, range of, 10–12
  normal joints, 17
Mucous membrane lesions, 14
Muscles, 4
  activity in posture control, 136
  muscle power
    assessing elbow joint, 58
    assessing hand, 66
    grading, MRC scale, *12*
  muscle wasting, 12
    knee joint, 100, 101, 102

shoulder girdle, 39
Myofascial pain, 71, *72*

Nail changes, 14
Neck
  examination, 76–79
    assessing movement, 78, *79*
  pain, 37
  see also Cervical spine
Nerve roots, 74, *75*
  root lesions, 38, 61, *75*, 83
  root stretching tests, 83, *84*
Neurological examination, 79, 81
Night pain, 6–7, 71
  shoulder, 38
Nodules, 13
  forearm, 55, 56
  hand, 63
Nottingham Health Profile, 26

Ober test, 93, 94
Olecranon
  bursitis, 54, 55, 56
    aspiration and injection, 60
  process, 55
Osgood-Schlatter's disease, 104, 109
Osteoarthritis
  clinical outcome measures, clinical
    trials, 27
  Doyle index, 24
  in hands, 64, *65*
  in knee, 99, 101
    attachment lesions, 109, 110
  radiological assessment, 25
  Western Ontario and McMaster
    Universities Osteoarthritis Index
    (WOMAC), 26
Osteochondritis, os tibialis, 119
Osteodystrophy, hypertrophic, 62, 64
Osteoporosis, 81
Ourcome Measurement in
  Rheumatoid Arthritis Clinical Trials
  (OMERACT)
    conference, 27
Outcome measures, 23, 25–26, 27
Oxalate, in synovial fluid, 152

Pain, general aspects, 5–7
  atypical, 62
  night pain, 6–7, 38, 71
  pain scales, 24
  psychogenic pain, 72
  referred pain, 6, 61, 71
  rest pain, 6
  screening questions, 16
  severe unremitting, 71
  soft-tissue, 71
  usage pain, 6, 10–11
Palmar erythema, 14
Pancoast's tumour, 36
Parkinson's disease, 142
Patellar
  abnormalities, 105
  apprehension test, 100
  ligament, 98
  position, 104–105
  subluxation, 100
  tap test, 102, *103*
Patellofermoral
  osteoarthritis, injection, 109, 110
  stress test, 22
Pelvic tilt, 90
Peripheral nerve involvement, 62
Peroneus muscle, testing, *125*
Pes cavus, 117
Pes planus, 115, 116–117, *119*
Phalen's sign, 69
Phantom pain, 62
Phrenic nerve irritation, 36
Physician global assessment, 25
Pigeon-toe, 117
Pinch grip test, 58, 59
Pivot shift test, 107
Planter fasciitis, 116
  injection, 127
Plantar flexion, assessing, 124
Plantar neuralgia, 115
Plicae, 4
Polydactyly, 115
Polymorphs, 151
Popliteus bursa, 104
Posterior cruciate ligament, 98
Posterior drawer test, knee joint, 107

Posture, 8, 136–139
  evolution of standing, 136
  examination, 137–139
    lower limb causes, abnormal
      posture, 138–139
  mechanisms of control, 136
  normal resting position, 16–17
  physiological sensory
    imbalance, 137
  sensory function, 136–137
  standing patient, 18, 19
  and walking development, 143
Power grip, 61
  testing, 20, 21
Precision
  grip, 61
  pinch, 21
Prepatellar bursa, 102, 103
  injection, 109, 110
Primary cartilaginous joints, 3, 4
Pronator teres syndrome, 59
Prone-lying test, 105, 106
Proximal myopathies, 142
Pseudoachondroplasia, 96
Psoas muscle, 74
  abscess, 74, 81
Psoriasis, hands, 64, 65
Psychogenic
  gait disturbance, 18
  pain, 72
Pterygoid muscles, palpation, 132

Q-angle, 104, 105
Quadriceps femoris, 98
Quadriceps lag, 105
Questionnaires
  health assessment
    questionnaires, 26
  pain scales, 24
  quality of life assessments, 12

Radia nerve, 68
  lesions, 69
    radial tunnel syndrome, 53
Radioisotope injections, 147
Radiological assessments, 25
  shoulder joint, 48

temporomandibular joint, 134
Radioulnar joints, palpation, 57
Ragocytes, 151
Red eye, 14
Referred pain, 6
  hand, 61
  spine, 71
Reflex algodystrophy, 62
Reiter's cells, 151
Repetitive strain injury, 62
Resisted active (isometric)
  movement, 10, 11–12
Rest pain, 6
Retrocalcaneal bursitis, 116, 121
Rheumatoid arthritis
  articular indices, 24
  clinical outcome measures, clinical
    trials, 27
  in hands, 64, 65, 66
  health assessment
    questionnaires, 26
  palmar erythema, 14
  radiological assessment, 25
  steroid injections, 148
  toe deformities, 117, 118
Rice bodies, 151
Ritchie articular index, 24
Rotator cuff
  anatomy, 32, 33
  disorders, 31–32
    complete tears, 47, 48
    pain radiation, 37, 38, 46
    tendinitis, 37, 38

Sacral vertebrae, 72, 74
Sacroiliac joints, 85
'Sausage' toes, 116
Scapula
  rotation, 35
  'winging', 40
Scapulothoracic bursitis, 40
Scheuermann's disease, 80
Schirmer tear test, 14
Sciatic stretch test, 83
'Scissor-like' gait, 142
Scleritis, 14
Scoliois, 80

leg length discrepancy, 139
Secondary cartilaginous joints, 4
Semimembranosus
  bursa, 104
  muscle, 98
Semitendinosus, 98
Sensory ataxia, 142
Sepsis, erythema, 8
Serratus anterior palsy, 39, 40
Sesamoiditis, 120
Shoulder joint, 31–50
  anatomy, 32–35
    additional structures
      around, 33–34
    blood supply, 34
    functional anatomy, 35–36
    joint capsule, 32
    muscles around shoulder, 32–33
    nerve supply, 34, 35
  aspiration and injection, 48–50
  clicking sensation, 39
  crepitus, 38
  developmental abnormalities,
    35
  dislocation, 36, 39
  evolution, 35
  examination, 20, 39–48
    inspection, 39–40
    muscle testing and range of
      movements, 40–43, 44
    pain on movement, 43, 44, 45,
      46, 47
    palpation, 40
  investigations, 48
  pain, 31
    general history, 36–37
    occupational history, 37
    pain history, 37–38
    pain spots, injection, 50
  stiffness, 38
  weakness, 38, 47
Sicca syndrome, 14
Sickness Impact Profile, 26
Skin changes, 8–9
  hands, 63
Sleep disturbance, 7
Slipped femoral epiphysis, 86

Soft-tissue
   injection around knee, 109–111
   pain, 71
Spasticity, 142
Speed's test, 44, *45*
Spinal cord, 75
Spine, 71–85
   embryological development, 3
   examination, 76–85
      gait disturbance, 17
      quick screen, 85
   functional anatomy, 72–75
      blood supply, 74
      ligaments, 74
   movement, *75, 76*
   pain patterns, 71–72
Spondylolisthesis, 81, 83
Sprengel's shoulder, 35
Spurling's manoeuvre, 79
Staggering gait, 142
Stamping gait, 142
Standing patient, inspection, 18–21
   load line, 139
Sternoclavicular joint, 35, 36
   assessing stability, 40
   injection, 50
   pain, 37
   swelling, 40
Sternocleidomastoid, testing, 78
Sternomanubrial joint, injection, 50
Steroid injection, 147
   choice of needle, 149
   complications, 148
   contraindications, 147
   crystalline corticosteroids, 152
   dosage, 149
   follow-up advice, 149
   indications, *148*
   precautions, 149
   procedure, 148–149
   'steroid boost' effect, 108
Stiffness, 7
   knee joint, 99
   measurement of duration, 24
Straight leg raising test, 83, *84*
Stress pain, 10, *11*
Stress tests, *11*

Stretch reflexes, 136
Structural locking, posture
   control, 136
Subacromial bursa, 33, 36
Subcutaneous bursae, 4
Subscapularis muscle, 33
Subtalar joint, 113, 136
   aspiration and injeciton, 125, 126
   testing, 122, *123*
Sudek's atrophy, 62
Superior radioulnar joint, 52
Supinator muscle, 53
Suprascapular nerve, 34, 35
   entrapment, 38
Supraspinatus muscle, 32, 33
   injection, 49
   testing, 42, 43, *45*
   wasting, 39
Supraspinatus tendon, complete
   tear, *44*
Swan neck deformity, 8, *66*
Sweating, loss of, 63
Swelling, 7, *9–10*
   around shoulder, 40
Synarthroses, 3–4
Synchondrosis, 3
Syndactyly, 115
Syndesmosis, 3
Synovial fluid, 4
   aspiration, 147
      choice of needle, 149
   examination, 149, 150–153
      cell count and differential, 151
      conventional light
         microscopy, 151
      general aspects, collection and
         storage, 150
      gram stain and culture, 152–153
      macroscopic
         appearance, 150–151, plate 1
      polarised microscopy, 151–152
      special tests, 153
Synovial joints, 4
   classification, *5*
Synovial membrane, 4
Synovitis, signs, 8, 9, *11*
   muscle wasting, 12

range of movement limitation,
   10
Systemic illness, symptoms, 7
Systemic lupus erythematosus,
   hands, *64*
Systemic sclerosis, hands, *64*

Talipes, 115
   congenital talipes equinovarus,
      143
   talipes equinus, 115, 117
Talocalcaneo-navicular joint, 113
Tarsal tunnel syndrome, 115,
   116
   injection, 127
Teeth, inspection, 133
Temporalis muscle, palpation, 132
Temporomandibular joint, 128–135
   additional tests, 134
   anatomy, 128–129
      functional anatomy, 129
   developmental abnormalities, 130
   examination, 20, 131–134
      inspection, 131
      muscle and neurological
         examination, 133
      palpation, 131–132
      range of motion, 132–133
   history, 130
   injection, 134–135
   phylogenetic
      development, 129–130
   symptoms, 130–131
Temporomandibular joint (*Cont.*)
   temporomandibular pain
      syndrome, 130, 133, 134
Tenderness, 10, 71
Tendonosis, 120
Tendons, 4
Tennis elbow *see* Lateral epicondylitis
Tenosynovitis
   ankel extensors, 116
   de Quervain's, 54, 66
      Finkelstein's test, *11*, 12, *66*
   posterior tibial tendon,
      injection, 127
   signs, 10, *11*

Teres minor, 32, 33

Therapeutic aspiration, 147

Thigh circumference, measuring, *102*

Thomas' test, 92–93

Thompson articular index, 24

Thoracic outlet syndrome
    Adson's manoeuvre, 79
    pain radiation, 38
    tests, 46

Thoracic spine
    anatomy, 72, 73, *74*
    examination, 80–81

Thoracolumbar scoliosis, 80

Thumb, 61
    movements, 66, 67
        adductor weakness, *68*
        osteoarthritis, carpometacarpal
            joint, 65
        Z deformity, 66

Thyroid, examination, 76, 77, 78

Tibial bowing, 101

Tibiofibular joint, 107–108
    distal, 112

Tibiotalar joint, 112

Tinel's sign, 58, 69

Toe-in gait, 117

Torticollis, 78

Trapezius
    testing, 78
    wasting, 39

Treacher Collins syndrome, 130

Tremor, 62–63

Trendelenburg
    gait, 18, 90, 142
    test, 91

Triamcinolone hexacetonide, 148
    crystals, synovial fluid, plate 9
    dosage, 149

Triangle sign, 56, *57*

Triceps, 52, *53*

Trochanteric bursa, 88
    bursitis, 88, *89*, 92
        injection, 95

Ulnar nerve lesions
    entrapment, 56, 58
    features, *68*, 69

Valsalva manoeuvre, 79

Vastus medialis obliquus, 98

Vertebrae, 72–73, *74*

Vertigo, 137

Visual analogue scale (VAS), 24

Volkmann's contracture, *69*

Waddling gait, 18, 90, 142

'Waiter's arm' deformity, 68

Walking *see* Gait

Warmth, inflammation assessment, 9

'Weaver's bottom' *see* Ischiogluteal
    bursa: bursitis

Western Ontario and McMaster
    Universities Osteoarthritis Index
    (WOMAC), 26

World Health Organisation
    (WHO), 23

Wright's manoeuvre, 46

Wrist, 61, 64
    bones, 63–64
    nerve supply, 68

Yergason's test, 44, *45*

Z deformity of thumb, 66

Ziehl-Neelson stain, 152